ONE LUM
OR TWC

GEORGE WALKER, M.B.E.

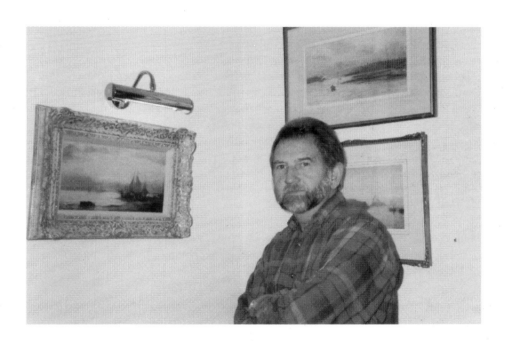

NEWCASTLE UPON TYNE, 2001

1

Acknowledgements

As with my first book it is impossible to mention everyone I have known and come to know in my now 14 year battle against cancer - the list would be endless. They all know, however, how much they have all come to mean to me and how much I appreciate their love and their friendship.

I have already dedicated this book to my family and the RVI medical team in appreciation of everything they have done for me and wish them to know how very important that has been to me.

The continuation and the great success of the North East Last Night of the Proms is a great tribute to the marvellous people who year after year have helped to produce it. They are, of course, Benjamin Luxon CBE, Janice Cairns, Sir Thomas Allen, Suzanne Manuell, Sheila (Luxon) Amit, Rachel Luxon, Bradley Creswick, Blake Fisher, James Cleverton, Richard Bloodworth, David Haslam, Len Young, Northern Sinfonia and Newcastle and Ryton Choral Societies - what a wonderful team.

To my friends Barry Latham, Ian Turner, Peter Allan OBE, Alan Young & Russell Slaymaker, who, as Directors & Trustees, help us to keep NEPAC Charity Trust "on the road" - thank you for your help.

Regarding this book, I owe a great debt of thanks to Jackie Danskin, who has typed my many thousands of words and helped me link together all the various chapters, written in many cases out of context; Rosalynde for reading everything I've written and encouraging me to continue when sometimes I felt like giving up; Bernard Baxter OBE for reading the manuscript and telling me it was worth publishing and Ross Taylor CBE, whose persistent "nagging" and encouragement, ensured that, I started and didn't dare not finish this story!

To David and Jennifer Cranston, who have unstintingly helped Rosalynde & me with concert work during the past two years when I have struggled with health problems - a huge thank you to you both.

Finally, I am grateful to Tom Moffat MBE and Carole Shotton of Casdec Ltd. for helping me to publish and distribute the book in a very cost saving way to enable more of the proceeds to go to Cancer Research and for producing a book for me in such a delightful and interesting format.

*This book is
Dedicated
To*

*Rosalynde, Marc and Roxanne,
my wonderful family, who have shared
all my struggles to survive with
great love and devotion
and to
Professor Stephen J Proctor
and his "Team" of Doctors & Staff on Ward 8,
the Oncology Unit Staff (Ward 6a)
and the Haematology Centre Staff (Ward 6b)
who have, on more than one occasion,
saved my life and the lives of many, many others*

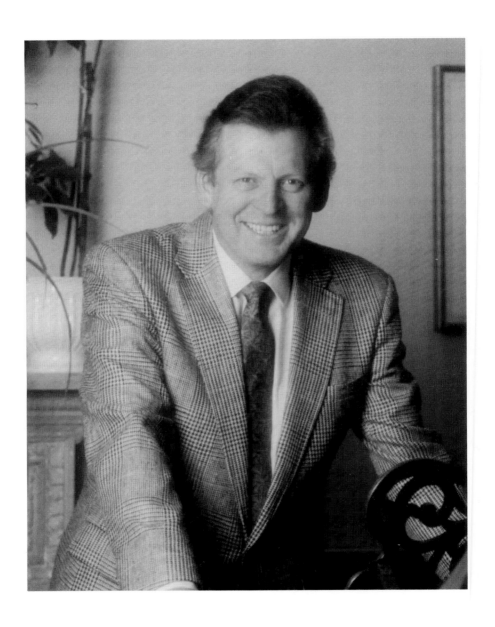

Photograph by Clive Barda Photography, London

Introduction
by Sir Thomas Allen, C.B.E.

George handed me his magnum opus to read at a time in my life when there wasn't a moment to be spared.

Rehearsals, flights, performances of opera and recital as well as getting together an exhibition of drawings and paintings. He then, as George will, set me a deadline, which brought me to my senses in realising that I had to set to with some serious reading.

As it turned out, that was no ordeal.

The first chapters flew by as I recognised the descriptions so well of the young boy burgeoning into the young man into the fumbling young lover and the inescapable school conflict that follows.

Just a few years later than George describes, exactly the same dilemmas were happening to myself and no doubt several million other teenagers.

What is it about George?

The quick answer would be Ros.

To meet them is to know them is to love them is to work for them.

Today it's rare to find this wonderful closeness of family and friends that they enjoy. It is something to behold.

Enthusiasm is the credo of the Walker household and in their company it becomes very infectious.

We all benefit from their being and their love and I am glad to have made time in my mad life for The North East Proms, George and Ros and for this second book in George's rich life.

The book is great, I felt so comfortable with it recognising the fine North East feel to it.

Here's strength to your elbow, George, and all those other unpleasant bits that give you gyp from time to time.

Many many many congratulations on your MBE Award - it has never been more well deserved and couldn't have gone to an nicer "feller".

Tom.

"One Lump or Two?"

A Sequel to "Cancer is Only a Word" (1994)
By George Walker, M.B.E.

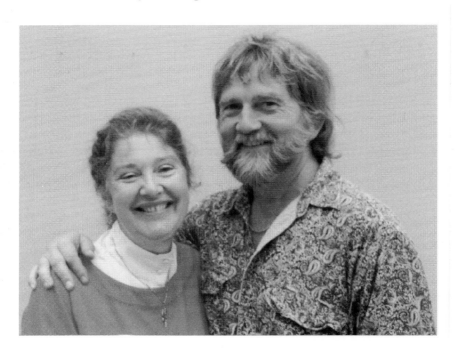

Foreword
Why a Sequel?

T he date is Tuesday 19th May 1998, nothing very spectacular about it except that the weather is glorious and I have just made an important decision after Rosalynde recounted a phone call she had with Professor Steve Proctor while I was in Newcastle. Strangely enough the seed for this decision was sown last Saturday when I called at a pretty, little garden centre called "Jan's Plants" at the small Northumberland village of Etal in North Northumberland. Jan's husband Jimmy has grown Kelso onions for years and he always keeps me a couple of boxes for our cottage garden and our garden at Westerhope near Newcastle.

After our usual friendly greetings and the question I have been asked more times than any other - "How are you George?". A question always asked with slight trepidation, which I readily sense but it is rewarding though to see the genuine sigh of relief when I say "I'm fine, thanks." Anyway, Jimmy then said, "I'm reading your book, 'Cancer is Only a Word' for the second time. I don't read all that much and usually it's just books for necessity like garden catalogues but yours is different. You have everything in your story - there's happy and sad bits; there's bits that make you laugh and bits that make you cry; there's bits that depress you and bits that lift you up. Why don't you write another one?"

I've been asked that on more than one occasion but I've always put it straight to the back of my mind partly because the amount of work involved but mainly because I haven't felt the urge or the need to do so. I also like books with happy endings and I couldn't be sure whether a sequel would have a happy ending. At this very moment and for the first time I feel both are possible. The story I am about to unfold more or less begins where the other left off. It will be written with the verbal warning that all the ingredients mentioned by Jimmy will appear again, but the strongest of them all will be that of hope sprinkled with humour as events lead up to the telephone call from Steve Proctor to Rosalynde

By the time the story nears completion the outcome of that phone call should also be revealed.

For people who did not have the opportunity to read my first book, "Cancer is Only a Word", which was published in 1994 and sold out relatively quickly for a book written by an unknown and totally inexperienced "author" it will help you to move on to the first chapter of this book if I gave a brief synopsis.

"Cancer is Only a Word" began as a diary of events, which overtook me around Easter 1988 when I found a large lump in my abdomen. This was eventually found to be non-Hodgkin's disease, a form of lymphoma which is a blood related cancer. Initially the disease was diagnosed as cancer of the pancreas and I was literally told I only had about 12 weeks to live. After a traumatic week of recovering from the biopsy and waiting for the final results, I was told it was lymphoma – I had been given a reprieve!

The "diary" was a form of therapy suggested to me by Rosalynde, my wonderful supportive wife, who has borne the burden of my illness with me for nearly 14 years, and it slowly turned into a book as one amazing thing after another took place during several recurrences of the disease. The title may sound arrogant but it was not meant to be; it was taken from a poem written by a teenager with cancer and I was very moved by her attempts to give the same inspirational message as do these following chapters. She is another success story, is now married with a family so for her cancer really was only a word.

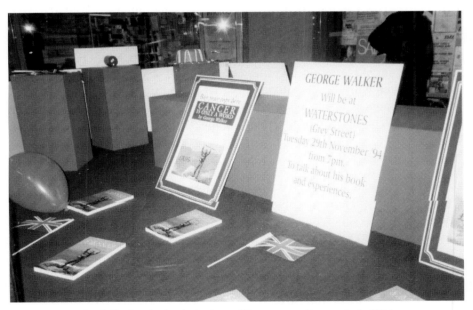

Book display for book signing at Waterstones, Newcastle in 1994

Chapter 1
The First Book

"Cancer is Only a Word" was launched at the 5th North East "Last Night of the Proms" in October 1994. Five years after starting to write it two thousand copies were printed and if it hadn't been for the generosity of Anne Flowers and the Newcastle Centre Library, who not only helped me with the publishing but very kindly allocated me storage space for the small mountain of boxes which arrived from the printers, Rosalynde and I would not have been able to move for books at our already overcrowded home (I'm a great collector of Victoriana much to Rosalynde's controlled annoyance).

Happily we sold over 300 copies at the concert which just left a mere 1700 to distribute and a few days later I launched myself into yet another career – book salesman and distributor extraordinaire.

My first real attempt actually took place in Penrith after the concert. We were on route to Borrowdale for a walking weekend – an idyllic escape from the hectic, energy sapping, build up to the concert. We stayed at High Lodore Farm, a place I'm loathe to mention because it's so good and I'm afraid all future readers will go flocking there. So Phyllis and Martin, prepare yourselves for the onslaught.

Armed with my brief case and a note pad serving as an order book, I walked into the first book shop we came across. It was actually one of those shops like John Menzies and WH Smith which sold a multitude of things as well as books. Not having a clue on how to begin I asked the assistant if I could speak to the Manager who appeared and listened to my somewhat hesitant sales spiel. She wasn't impressed but out of sympathy, rather than boosting her company's sales figures, offered to take one copy at 30% trade discount saying that if that sold she might consider taking another one or perhaps even two if I could drop them into the shop.

As I had already naively told her all the proceeds were for cancer research and patient care, I was taken aback at the amount of discount she was wanting and a round trip of about 150 miles to deliver additional copies would drain away any further income and my patience. I then tried to persuade her to review her order and discount but to no avail. So I beat a retreat without releasing a single copy. The weekend wasn't a sales disaster though because I met a couple of old friends from my school days in an antique shop in Penrith where I backed them into a corner and released them for a fee of ten pounds in return for which they received a signed copy. Phyllis and Martin bought a copy during our stay at their farm. Another of their residents brought the total to three before we finally departed full of good food and wine and feeling splendidly re-vigorated by the peace and beauty of the English Lake District.

One Lump or Two

Slowly but surely my sales and distribution experience improved and eventually, after many miles of driving around an area which stretched from North Shields to Hexham and Newcastle to Edinburgh, I managed to unload about a thousand books in shops ranging from the "real" book shops like Waterstone's and Dillon's to multi-purpose shops like WH Smith, newsagents and even garden centres where they experimented in garden gravel, sand and cement, tea rooms, children's play areas and the occasional plant thrown in.

My two "favourite" hospitals, the RVI and the Newcastle General sold a lot for me and I sent a hundred copies to the Bristol Cancer Centre as a gift for their kindness to me in 1988 when my world was in darkness.

Perhaps my proudest moment, when I actually felt I had written a book and had earned the title of "author" was when the Waterstone's branch at Newcastle asked me to do a book signing evening which I promptly accepted. The evening was advertised by Waterstone's and about 40 people turned up. Wine was served, I gave a talk about the book and my experiences and signed quite a few copies that night. Most of the people who turned up were, of course, friends and colleagues but it was another one of those memorable experiences that only happened because of cancer.

Four years on cancer has continued to leap in and out of my life with that strange mixture of unforgettable, happy and exhilarating oases of pleasure interspersed liberally with fear and depression.

The book itself has sold out but orders are still coming in and most of them from areas of the British Isles outside the north east. I have even had orders from Canada, America, Australia, Norway, Spain and, would you believe, Tokyo.

I've received many complimentary letters, some of them very moving. All of them express the fact that the book helped them in whatever situation they found themselves with cancer, whether as a sufferer or a carer; making it all very worthwhile for me.

What else came out of it from a number of the letters was the comment that although they had got to know me well as a person it was only really from around my 50th year onwards and they would have liked to have known more about me in my earlier years. The following chapters will hopefully make up for that and I've kept the sex, crime and violence down to a minimum!

Chapter 2
Early Childhood

L ife for me began on 3rd November in 1937 just before World War II exploded onto the scene. The word cancer was not in my early vocabulary, in fact it was rarely spoken out loud not just because the world I knew was hell bent on killing everyone by other means, but because the disease hadn't spread out its ugly tentacles quite so blatantly and people were very afraid of it.

I remember clearly as a child hearing the whispers, which went round the room, when someone near and dear or a neighbour up the road had succumbed to an unnamed illness. Words like "terrible pain","poor soul","he was just like a skeleton","You wouldn't have recognised her" would fall upon my inquisitive, young ears and I wondered with fear and trepidation what ghastly thing had struck down a fellow human being. I discovered later it wasn't just the disease, which frightened people,

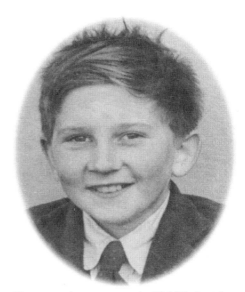

Me at a tender age - note the "fab" hair style

it was the word itself and it was never mentioned. I suppose the only one good thing we can thank cigarettes for is the way it dramatically brought the word into the public eye and mind but that was a long way into the future. Cigarette smoking was very fashionable then; the King, politicians, fighter pilots, film stars, everyone seemed to smoke in those days, except my mother and she lived to the ripe old age of 86. Pollution was virtually non existent or at least the world was not aware of the dangers then. Today some cancers can be cured and in some cases even prevented. The world is becoming increasingly aware of these facts and one day it will be wiped off the face of the earth.

Childhood can be a wonderful experience if you are fortunate enough to spend it amidst love and affection. The mind of a child sees life as it simply is, there's no place for unpleasantness unless it is forced upon it. A child too, is eager to learn but it thrives best on things which are interesting and exciting. Death and words like cancer are experienced but are quickly pushed to one side to be rediscovered amongst the approaching pitfalls and trials of adulthood.

One Lump or Two

My first experience of this very natural act was at primary school. We were asked to bring a penny to our form teachers for a collection to buy flowers for a schoolmate, who, as far as we were concerned, had just not come to school one morning. He wasn't in my close circle of friends but playground chatter enlightened me to the fact that his mother had gone to his bedroom to waken him for school and she couldn't rouse him. That wasn't so disturbing to our innocent minds. We missed him but we were not frightened by his abrupt departure. We, in our simplicity, associated death with sleep and our friend had just gone to sleep and hadn't woken up.

It hit me harder when, a few years later at junior school, a classmate died. This time I knew him well; I had sat beside him in class and we had played together. To make matters worse he died on my birthday and I found that very hard to take. I was older and wiser by this time and tried to find out what really happened. I experienced the sadness of it as well as a little fear because there were tragic circumstances involved. His parents had separated and it was his mother who had left home. He had been out playing and had been soaked to the skin, caught by the cold November rain. The result was a chill followed by pneumonia, which in those days sometimes proved fatal. I often wondered if his mother had been home would her maternal care have prevented the tragedy?

Today death is all around us more vividly than ever. Even though my childhood days were spent with a war raging around my ears, I honestly don't think we had the same exposure to it as we have now. Every form of mass communication seems to fling it at us. Films, television, newspapers and videos are the worst culprits and they even depict it "live" and I make no apology for the pun.

In the same breath, however, it is the same communications, particularly television, which have brought the word cancer well and truly out into the open. There I hope it will remain because only if we face it, hear it and speak it, especially alongside words like cure, success, remission, victory and so on, can we help rid ourselves of the fear and the awe we have of it.

Recently I read a letter from a friend whose daughter had died of skin cancer after a determined fight which lasted eleven years. In it he said:-

"It wasn't the quantity of life which was important to her, it was the quality. *She learned to live with the cancer not die from it.*"

Wonderful, moving words!

Chapter 3
School Days and Falling in Love
for the First Time

If I was granted one wish, which could change my life right from the beginning, I would ask for one thing above all else, a real talent. Oh, I am capable enough in many respects but deep down I know I am really just a survivor and it is only those strong basic instincts, which have managed to raise me from what could have been a very ordinary life. It must be wonderful to have a God-given natural talent especially one which brings pleasure to people like singing or playing a musical instrument.

At the moment of writing this, I am 60 years of age and it seems a long, long time ago since I was a child.

I was the fifth of six sons. My grandparents were a coal mining family on my father's side and railway engine driving on my mother's side; her father used to drive the Flying Scotsman during the wonderful days of steam. My father "clawed" his way out of the pits to become a shop assistant and then manager with the North Eastern Co-operative Society. My mother served her apprenticeship as a French Salon dressmaker at Fenwicks of Newcastle but followed the tradition of the day by never working again for a wage after her marriage. Her sewing skills were put to great use throughout her early marriage as she stitched, sewed and altered clothes to make sure we were all turned out clean and smart for school. We lived in a succession of five houses altogether but I can only remember two of them, the first of which had two bedrooms and two downstairs rooms, a large pantry with a sink in it and a small gas burner. The toilet was outside next to the coal house, across a brick yard, which was well below the level of the road and pavement. I used to hate climbing those steps to the gate and I don't really know why.

I loved the kitchen range with its black-leaded iron work and shiny brass rail, which for 364 days of the year had shirts, vests and towels hanging to dry on it but on one special day nothing else but socks, which were placed there on Christmas Eve with our letters to Santa Claus. In the morning we would find them filled with sweets, fruit and whatever my parents could afford at the time and on the table was an empty sherry glass with a drop still inside and a plate with a few crumbs of Christmas cake, telling us that Santa Claus had been visiting.

The range, too, was the main source of heat for the whole house but it had many more uses, the best of which was the food which came out of its oven and the big pan, which always seemed to be bubbling on the grate. Fresh bread, dumpling stew, leek pudding, blackberry and apple suet pudding, mince tarts, peas pudding, meat and "tatty" pie, were but a few of the mouth watering, stomach filling, north country savouries which were dished up for us by a much beleaguered but loving mum.

Constant hot water was available from the boiler in this multi-purpose range, as long as we could afford the coal to heat it. Wednesday and Sunday evenings were bath nights and the big tin bath was carried in from the yard with great ceremony and plonked in front of a roaring fire, even in summer. It was like a factory assembly line. Six naked, grubby lads fed in at one end by a critical mother and clean, shiny cherubs emerging at the other to be vigorously dried in front of the fire by a more impatient Dad, who was wanting to get off to the Club for a pint of beer with his friends.

Most of my stay at that house was spent in that living room, which is an apt name for it. I avoided the bedrooms like the plague and have only dim memories of sharing a huge bed with two of my brothers.

The front room as it was proudly called was only used on special occasions. It contained my mother's pride and joy in the way of furniture: record player or gramophone as it was called in those days, a chesterfield, two easy chairs, china cabinet and a coffee table. There was always a cold feel to this room except on those special occasions when the fire was lit and we could have tea from the best china. When we were ill and well enough to come down from the bedroom my mother would always light the fire and put us into this room. It made us feel special and well on the way to recovery.

When I was ten years old, our name finally came to the top of the council housing list and we moved to the other end of the town into a brand new 4-bedroomed council house with a very large piece of land. My mother promptly turned us all into slaves to make it a model garden, which the council officials gave due recognition in a letter which she proudly showed us.

The house seemed enormous but we filled it and I shared a bed with only one brother until National Service whipped two of them away and I became the possessor of my very own room.

By this time I was travelling 20 miles a day on a bus to Hexham where I attended the Queen Elizabeth 1 Grammar School. I failed the 11 plus exam or rather I gained what was called an "interview", which consisted of some aptitude tests and a real interview. This, I suppose, was with an education advisor or a teacher from the school. I don't think they were impressed with the books I read at the time, "Biggles" and "Just William" or my favourite radio programme "The Man in Black" narrated by Valentine Dyall, all about ghosts!

I then was fortunate though in having a new teacher, who believed that I had some ability and he encouraged me with my reading and writing and gave me extra maths to do at home. The best book I read then was "The Robe" by Lloyd C. Douglas. Years later I saw the film with Richard Burton playing the part of the centurion, who becomes so strangely affected by the robe Jesus wore prior to his crucifixion. It was a good film but did not leave the same impression as the book had done. Imagery from words are often more powerful and moving than seeing it on the screen.

My teacher's confidence in me was rewarded by my sitting the twelve plus examination and gaining a place at the Grammar School. They were wonderful years at Hexham Grammar School for Boys. Thankfully there was one for girls too and it was on the same site.

The only thing we shared , however, was the large hall which was entered at one end by the girls when they used it and at the other end by the boys. We walked up the hill to the school on opposite sides of the road and descended it in the same way at the end of the day. This itself wasn't a school rule but we were very shy of each other in the early years. As we moved towards fifth and sixth forms these barriers were broken and it was easy to see who was seeing who, just by watching the flow to and from school.

My first two years were very hard academically and I was usually to be found at or near the bottom of the class. The problem being that I was a year behind everyone else and subjects like algebra, geometry, physics and French were very hard to pick up while people were racing away from you. I shone though at Latin because it was only introduced in the second year and we all started at the same time.

I had my first real experience of love in those days. Our school bus travelled through a place called Riding Mill and one day I noticed a girl boarding the bus from there. Time just stood still, the bus went quiet or so I thought, except for the pounding of my heart and I stared at the back of her head all the way to Hexham. Every now and then she would turn her head to speak to her companion and I thought she had the most beautiful profile I had ever seen. That girl caused me to have rare moments of intense pleasure on the few occasions she let me take her out but hours and hours of heartache when she ignored my very existence. I used to day dream about her and try every means possible to see her during the school day to get her to notice me. I was desolate if, for some reason, she wasn't on the school bus in the morning and that was frequently because there were two buses on that route and it depended on which one arrived at her stop first; I would then have to wait for the 4pm bus home to see her again.

It took me a long time to get her out of my system. It's true you never really forget your first love. I still remember the pain and the pleasure I received from it.

One occasion when she allowed me to take her out to the pictures at Hexham, I suddenly realised I had gone overboard with sweets and ice cream and would not have enough money to get us both home - her to Riding Mill and me to continue to Prudhoe seven miles further on. I cursed myself for getting carried away and stupidly trying to make a big impression. The answer was simple, just tell her that I had ran out of money and did she mind paying for her own fare home. However, pride comes before a fall because I couldn't bring myself to do it. I didn't want to blow the chance I had of going steady with her. So, as all great lovers, I made the supreme sacrifice and with the last of my money I bought two tickets to Riding Mill. She turned as I gave the money to the conductor.

"Aren't you going straight home?" she said innocently.

"No", said the gallant idiot "I thought I'd walk you home and catch the next bus to Prudhoe."

She smiled put her arm through mine and my heart soared.

Half an hour later I stood beside her at the garden gate to her home and we kissed in the dark. It was marvellous, my legs were like jelly. "I'll see you on the bus tomorrow morning." I whispered and watched her walk up the garden path and into her house. Two and a half hours later I knocked at our door back at Pudhoe to be greeted by angry but very concerned parents, who were worried and upset at my extreme lateness.

I climbed into bed that night footsore and weary but with my pride intact and memories of those kisses at the garden gate.

I wonder what she's doing now and whether she ever thinks of the lad from Prudhoe, who was one of the first Grammar School boys to have a crewe cut, was caned for smoking after being caught having his first cigarette, who left school at the end of lower sixth to go into the R.A.F. to try and be a pilot and whose heart she broke on more than one occasion.

Apart from a disastrous love life, my teenage years were not terribly exciting. I wasn't really a rebel and didn't cause any trouble but I found, like the rest of my friends, that the illicit attraction of under-age drinking was irresistible.

I actually liked beer and enjoyed the excitement of trying to pass off as an over 18 year old. This only began when I was 17 years old and in the Lower VI so it was a really short-lived process. I never ventured into a pub in Prudhoe where I lived, it was always in Hexham and on a Saturday night when we all met up.

It was a ritual really, we all had about 5 shillings pocket money to spend (that's 25 pence by present standards). It was possible in the 50s to have a good night out on that amount and still have change. Unbelievable but it's true!

The ritual was the bus to Hexham, usually about 6 of us, straight into one of the pubs we knew would accept us, have a round or two (always halves – makes the money last) then on to another pub and so on. Eventually, merrier than when we started, we would end up at the Queen's Hall, one of two dance halls in Hexham. This was usually about 9.30 pm leaving us an hour to dance or ogle the girls or both. None of us was a great dancer and so it was more often than not ogling the girls but we all took part without fail in the "Bradford Barn Dance". This was usually just before 10 o'clock. We had to watch the clock

The Prudhoe Lads (and one lass)

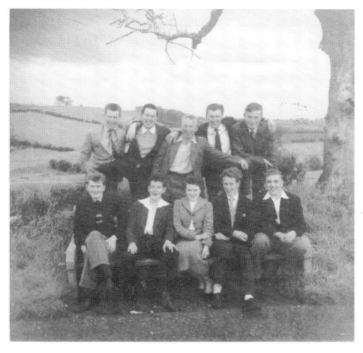

during this dance because the last bus left for Prudhoe at 10.30 pm. It was usually a sprint through the back streets to catch it in time.

One evening we almost failed but the outcome of that particular night was another long walk to Prudhoe and nothing to do with girls or dancing this time.

The "Prudhoe lads" as we were known caught the 10.30 pm last bus from Hexham. We were all worse for wear (half a dozen pints I think – really hardened drinkers!). I vaguely remember that it stopped at a bus stop. Chris Tyson, who was in a bad way, stood up and staggered down the aisle. Quite naturally we all thought the bus had arrived at Prudhoe and, like a bunch of sheep, we followed him off the bus in the same shuffling, head down, sorry for oneself, slightly sobering up way that late Saturday night "revellers" do.

We re-grouped on the pavement as the bus drove away into the cold, dark night and then watched stupefied as Chris proceeded to vomit copious amounts of beer into the hedgerow. A tiny ray of light began to filter through as the hedgerow should have been shops and I realised we were in the wrong place. We swivelled round in all directions trying to identify our position and realised we had dismounted at Corbridge – 8 miles from Prudhoe. The only way home was on "Shank's Pony", which I think is a lovely expression, and after many curses thrown at Chris and with no sympathy for his predicament, we set off on a long, shambling, miserable walk home.

The following Saturday saw us back in business though as if the incident had never happened – do we learn from our mistakes? Not really, not until we are too old and by then we want to relive them all again but cannot.

Chapter 4
National Service and Westminster College

After "O" Levels I had decided to stay on for "A" Levels partly because I still wanted to be near my elusive first love and partly because I really did love the school. My ambition had always been to fly, sparked off I suppose from the glamour of the Battle of Britain days. It was glamorous to us children but a horrific reality to those who lost their lives or were badly injured in it.

I did very well in the lower sixth but towards the end of it my heart wasn't really in the subjects I was studying. I have a practical rather than an academic mind and felt instinctively that I wasn't university material.

I had become very close to my English tutor, who had encouraged my interest in drama and who had persuaded me to join his Hexham Drama Group after seeing me perform as Raina Petkoff in our school production of Bernard Shaw's "Arms and the Man". A strange fact of life then, boys having to do the girls' parts when there was a school of willing girls "next door". I did, however, enjoy the Art Master's beautiful wife showing me how to put on a padded bra during the dress rehearsal and following performances.

Mr Alan Brown, or "Squirrel" as he was affectionately called because of his red hair, gave me some good, solid advice, "If you really want to go into the R.A.F," he said, "Go straight for your National Service, you can still try for air crew and if you make the grade you can sign on as a regular. If you are unsuccessful then you are only committed to two years, which you have to do anyway. What else have you thought about doing?". Before I could answer he said the words that were to plant a seed, which eventually grew to fulfilment.

"I think you would make a good teacher. You have an outgoing personality and you get on well with most people".

I'd never thought about teaching and had not done any background research into it. Careers advice was not a high profile in preparation for work in those days. It was usually university, the teaching profession, civil service at executive level, customs and excise etc. or a commission in the Armed Forces on offer then. This highlights how inadequate careers guidance was in those days.

"Squirrel" told me all about Colleges of Education, that it was a three year course and it enabled you to teach in Primary, Junior or Secondary Schools at whatever age group you preferred. My "O" levels were good enough to get me a place and he recommended his old college where he had done his teacher training as a post-graduate after completing his English degree. "I know the Principal very well," Squirrel continued, nourishing the seeds he had planted. "I'm sure he would find you a place in two years' time. It's a super college right in the heart of London and with a great sporting tradition. You've just got your rugby and cricket colours, they will stand you in good stead."

I thanked him and said I would think about it.

"Talk it over with your parents" were his parting words, "They'll be able to get a grant to cover your fees and expenses."

Suddenly from that conversation my future was secured. I don't know where you are "Squirrel", or whether you are still alive, you must be well over 70 years old now but you have my heartfelt thanks and gratitude for giving me your wisdom and advice all those years ago. Please forgive me for sometimes being a right little so and so in your lessons during the years, playing the fool instead of soaking up the richness of what you were trying to teach us. Thank you, too, for seeing something in me which no one else did.

Events raced away from me from that moment. My parents supported the idea. "Squirrel" was true to his word and wrote to the Principal of Westminster College on my behalf. Just before the end of the summer term of 1955 I set off on my very first trip to London to be interviewed for a place in his college. That was an adventure in itself; country boy goes to the big city! I did it all in one day. A round trip of 600 miles by bus, train and tube.

I was terrified by the momentous step I was taking into the world and awed by the size and the vigour of London. At the end of the day I was very proud of my achievement. The only mistake I made was ending up at the famous Westminster Public School instead of Westminster College; although I found out later that Westminster College was one of the top colleges for teacher training in the country.

The college itself was a lovely old building, which seemed as though London had been built around it. It was cloistered and ivy covered and when I stepped through the great wooden door into the quadrangle, the noise and bustle of London were shut out as the door closed behind me.

The Principal, The Reverend H. Trevor-Hughes M.A., was also a Methodist Minister but wasn't bothered by the fact that a confirmed Anglican had applied to attend a Methodist College. He was a mild, gentle man whose inner core of steel was not apparent until the day he suspended me from the college for slipping away home to see Rosalynde a day earlier than I should have done at half term. I would have got away with it but Ben Luxon and my other friends did exactly the same thing without saying a word to me! We sat together in Chapel and created a very noticeable gap on the morning we all slipped away. We attended Chapel everyday as part of college life and it was a good way to keep an eye on people.

I liked the Principal from the start and continued to do so throughout my college days. A week after my return from the interview in London, I shakily opened the envelope with the college crest stamped on it and read that he was pleased to offer me a place from September 1957 after conscription in the Armed Forces.

One Lump or Two

National Service did not bother me as much as it might have done. Two of my elder brothers had already served their time, one in Egypt, and they had both enjoyed it. Another brother was in the Royal Navy training to be an engineering officer so it seemed a natural step to take. I was eager to try for aircrew, which made it more a voluntary act than one of conscription.

I was in for a culture shock and no mistake!

As a 17 year old schoolboy I left Hexham Grammar School in July 1955, and put five happy years behind me. Eight weeks later my father's fifth son became a man.

It began outside a draughty railway station in a god-forsaken place called Cardington whilst carrying a battered, old suitcase containing all my worldly goods. Milling all around me were other young lads looking equally bewildered and carrying similar suitcases. Suddenly, 3 blue-grey lorries appeared out of the darkness and stopped in the station car park. Alien creatures in uniform jumped down and proceeded to stamp around us, screaming and bawling at the top of their voices. Everything had to be done at the double. We were herded like sheep towards the lorries where we climbed up and disappeared into the canvas covered awning still clutching our belongings.

We clung to the bench seats as the lorries raced us to our destination. My mind was in a whirl. My brothers hadn't prepared me for this sort of introduction.

All I can remember after that was arriving at Cardington R.A.F. Station, jumping down from the wagons and being rushed into a huge hangar where they gave us sheets, blankets and pillows, knife, fork, spoon and mug. From there we were taken to barrack blocks and allocated a bed, bed space and a locker. We dumped our things and rushed back outside to be taken on the double to the cookhouse for supper. Some of the lads had forgotten their utensils in the panic and were bawled at by the duty cooks, who then grudgingly flung some spares onto their trays for them. Back in the barracks we made our beds as best we could, unpacked our things and climbed miserably into bed wondering what the next day had in store for us.

I could write a book about my National Service days. Suffice to say that once I got over the trauma of the first days, I enjoyed

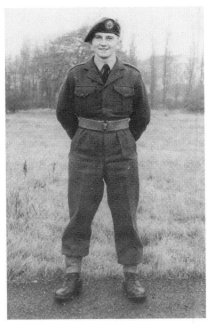

Me, as a "Sprog" at "square bashing" at R.A.F. Padgate, Lancashire

20

Me with my Signals Team towards the end of National Service

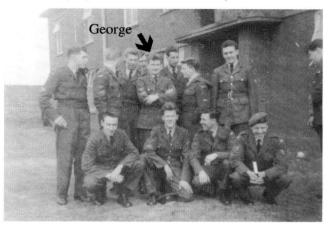

the life very much. I even enjoyed my eight weeks of "square bashing" at Padgate in Lancashire although that too was a shock to my system. I did, however, learn discipline and to look after myself in more ways than one. I learned too about comradeship and to appreciate home and my family, who supported me through the lonely times with letters and parcels. There isn't any real substitute for National Service these days and I often think the modern youngster would benefit a great deal from that sort of experience.

I never made aircrew because of perforated ear drums from some serious childhood illness which probably explains my oncoming deafness now. I was told that I was officer material but would have to sign on as a regular. If I couldn't fly then I wanted to teach and that is how things turned out. Before I left National Service though, I did reach the dizzy heights of full Corporal, which was quite an achievement for a National Serviceman. I spent my last year in charge of an underground telecommunication installation at 13 Group Headquarters. This really was nothing more than a fairly big telephone and teleprinter exchange but it played a role in communications between all the other R.A.F. Stations in the Group and the outside world and gave me invaluable administration experience.

Before I left National Service, a very important meeting took place which changed my life and very much for the better. I met my future wife, Rosalynde, who has stuck by me through thick and thin, for better or for worse ever since and who, I'm really glad to say, is still beside me. Why I deserve that honour I'm not really sure as I have my moments!

Met is probably the wrong word to use, met again is a more accurate description. Rosalynde lived at a place I hadn't even seen then called Haltwhistle. It is fifteen miles west of Hexham on the way to Carlisle. It just scrapes into Northumberland, which was why she ended up at Hexham Grammar School at the same time as me. Rosalynde was classed as one of the beauties by us budding experts on women and many of the boys fancied her. She was one of the girls we all liked to watch playing tennis especially as she possessed a very eye catching 34" bosom. She was not for me, however, as she had been snapped up very quickly by the good looking Romeo of the school and they seemed to have a steady courtship going. I wasn't over distressed by that as I was still brooding over my lost love but that doesn't mean I didn't notice her and admire her looks and personality.

By some strange quirk of fate I was on a weekend's leave towards the end of my R.A.F. days and decided to go to a dance at Hexham on the Saturday night and meet up with some of my old school friends. I went in uniform, of course, flaunting my Corporal's stripes and marksman's badge and had a really good time at the dance at the Royal Hotel.

I had to leave early to catch the last bus home to Prudhoe at 10.30p.m. and was moving from the cloakroom to the main exit when a lovely, young girl appeared in front of me. She was wearing an off the shoulder dance dress and looked vaguely familiar but there was something different about her, which I couldn't fathom.

She said, "Hello, it's George Walker isn't it?" and I recognised her voice immediately. It was Rosalynde without her beautiful ponytail, which she wore when we were at school. I think I preferred her ponytail but that didn't matter, she looked very attractive with short hair and I fell in love with her at that very moment.

I only had a few minutes to talk to her as I didn't want to walk to Prudhoe from Hexham but I managed to pluck up courage to ask her if I could get in touch with her again and perhaps have a game of tennis together. I was pleasantly surprised when she agreed and gave me her address and telephone number. I thought a lot about her after that meeting and eventually telephoned her and we had that game of tennis, which I let her win. You have to get your priorities right during courtship and use every ploy at your disposal!

Rosalynde had just finished her first year at Sunderland College of Education. She, too, wanted to be a teacher and she was very interested to hear that I was soon to start my training at Westminster. We went out together to the cinema at Hexham when I was next on leave and when I took her to the bus station to see her off, I gave her a "minto" sweet and after she had put it in her mouth, said to her, "I've never kissed a girl with a sweet in her mouth before". How original can one be but it worked and we had our first kiss.

Soon after that I left for a months' fire fighting course to an aerodrome at Moreton in the Marsh in the Cotswolds. The powers that be reckoned that if there was another war most of the time would be spent putting out fires after the holocaust so that is what we trained for prior to departure from National Service.

I was lovesick throughout that month and thought about Rosalynde everyday. I wrote a couple of letters and was thrilled when she replied to them. Looking back now I don't think our romance would have blossomed into the lifetime relationship it became if it hadn't been for another quirk of fate on a rugby pitch at Wembley (not the Wembley!) about two months after I started college in

London.

We continued writing but things seemed to be cooling off because of the distance and the commitments to our courses, which were very demanding. I was picked to play for the college first team along with a fellow from Cornwall called Ben Luxon. We had met soon after college began and took an instant liking to each other. He, too, had been in the R.A.F. and had actually been at R.A.F. Padgate when I was there. We were both keen on sport and had a mutual love of tennis. Not surprisingly we chose Physical Education as our second subject. My first was Geography and Ben's was English at the beginning but he quickly switched to Music when it became obvious that he had a superb, baritone, singing voice and loved music.

My debut for the first team put me into hospital with a suspected fractured skull. All I can remember was tackling an opponent, who was coming at me with the ball at one hell of a speed. Next thing, I woke up in a Wembley hospital blinking at a very pretty nurse peeling off my bloody and muddy shirt, shorts and underpants. She then proceeded to wash me and I watched in horror as I developed an erection, which under different circumstances, I would have been proud to achieve. Fortunately, she just carried on as though nothing had happened and I quickly shut my eyes to avoid further embarrassment. I must have closed them tightly because she said in a very sweet voice, "You can open them now, I've finished". Everyone today knows me with a beard and that was where I first grew it but only because I didn't have anything with me at the hospital to use for shaving.

I was kept there for two weeks but not because of the erection! Fortunately there was no fracture but severe concussion, which resulted one night in the worst nosebleed I have ever experienced. I had been told to lie still for a few days and suddenly felt as though I was drowning. I sat up quickly and blood shot out of both nostrils and mouth, all over the bedclothes. Nurses arrived very quickly but couldn't stop it and they sent for a doctor. I thought I was going to bleed to death but they eventually cauterised it, which was not very pleasant. First they stuck a needle up my nose and gave me a local anaesthetic, which froze my face. Then they pushed what looked like a soldering iron up both my nostrils. I could hear a sizzling noise and watched, horrified, as smoke drifted out of my nose and curled its way to the ceiling. I've never had a nose bleed since.

At the end of my hospital stay they sent me home to Northumberland to convalesce for three weeks. It was during that time that our relationship grew into mutual love as I was able to see Rosalynde frequently with Sunderland only about twenty miles from my home. I lost five valuable weeks at college including my first teaching practice and once again I found myself struggling to keep up with my fellow students.

College days were some of the happiest days of my life. London was a marvellous place to be based as a student. It turned out that Ben and I were very much in the minority as ex National Servicemen because it was being phased out. Most of the students were eighteen year olds straight from school. We stood out like sore thumbs as far as mature men of the world were concerned. I think we turned out better teachers, too, because we were much more street wise than the school lads. We were also much better at looking after ourselves, washing clothes, ironing and so on. Once, my first year flatmate, Harry from Rochdale, decided all our underpants were looking grey rather than their original white. He hit upon the bright idea of bleaching them. This seemed reasonable, so our group of six, which included Ben, who had all become close friends and shared three rooms adjacent to each other, handed over all our underpants except, fortunately, those we were wearing! Harry was straight from school and didn't realise the power of Domestos, which he borrowed from the cleaners' cupboard. He came back from the bathroom about an hour later with a large bucket of pulpy grey mush, which he had even stirred. I carefully dipped a ruler into the bucket and fished around. I lifted out what was left of a pair of underpants - the elastic waistband! Even the ruler started to dissolve.

The three years went by very quickly until one day I found myself once again saying good-bye to a bunch of great friends with whom I had shared some great experiences. We had shared each others' trials and tribulations and soon would be facing between 30 or 40 kids not much younger than ourselves but separated by the gulf between teacher and pupil. The exception was Ben who had been offered a place at the London Guildhall School of Music for further musical studies. It was a sadder moment than the end of my National Service. The bond of studentship had been closer than that of servicemen probably because there was more purpose to what we were doing and our aims were the same.

We promised to keep in touch and departed for the very different parts of England from whence we came. Of the six of us now, one became a world famous opera star, one is a college lecturer, one is a Headmaster, one is Head of a large Art Department, one is dead from a heart attack and I am the only one who developed cancer.

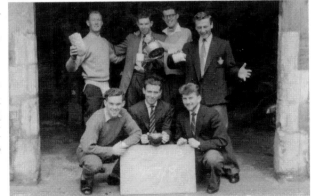

Our Brew Club at Westminster College,
Ben is wearing the "Jock Strap"!

Chapter 5
Benjamin Luxon, CBE

At this point many people who read the first book and, hopefully, this sequel will know Benjamin Luxon, the famous Cornish baritone, and I am sure they and any other classical music and opera lover would be interested to know how he managed to get started on the rocky road to fame and fortune.

I am really proud to say I was there to witness how it all began.

Ben had a good voice, we all knew that and we often "cashed" in on this with free beers when Ben started playing the piano and singing in our local college pub. He also influenced me and our small group of friends in our thoughts about music. He had a portable gramophone and some old 78s, which he was always playing and one of them in particular never seemed to be off the turntable. Robert Merrill and Jussi Bjorling singing the Pearl Fishers' Duet from Bizet's Opera, "The Pearl Fisher" – wonderful stuff.

He persuaded us to go to the opera, an incredible experience for me at that stage in my life. We used to walk to Covent Garden, join the queue for the "gods" and watch wonderful operas, albeit from a dizzy height, such as La Boheme, The Flying Dutchman, Tosca and one in particular, an operetta really, called "Die Fledermous" by Johan Strauss, with which I fell in love. If someone needs to be introduced to opera and operetta then my

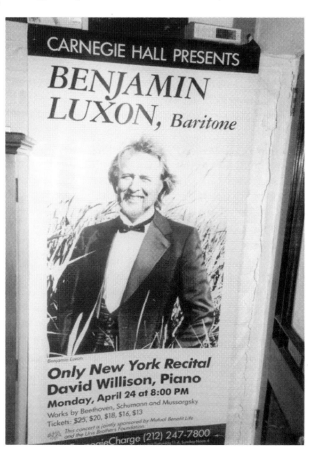

Poster of Ben Luxon at Carnegie Hall, New York

25

choice would be that one. Years later Rosalynde, our children, the Luxon family and I sat in a box at Covent Garden Opera House and watched Ben sing one of the leading roles in it with Kiri Te Kanawa and Herman Prey. The conductor for that special evening was none other than Placido Domingo, the world famous tenor, who we met afterwards at a dinner. I say "special" because it was New Year's Eve 1974 and the whole opera was being televised throughout Britain and Europe. Ben was at the pinaccle of his career. Before that, however, he had a long, hard and very steep hill to climb.

Our college music society often organised musical evenings and occasionally used Ben as an entertainer. Shortly after our evening of "Die Fledermaus" I saw a notice on the board that Marion Studholme, the famous soprano from Covent Garden, was to be a guest at the music society's next musical soiree and below that in small letters was "with Benjamin Luxon in support". She had sung in the performance of "Die Fledermaus" we had been to see. I asked Ben about this and he said they had asked him to sing a couple of songs to give Ms Studholme a break in the programme as she was also going to talk about her career and the world of opera as well as sing herself.

I didn't normally go to these evenings as they were a bit highbrow for my taste but this one was different because I'd seen her sing and I always enjoyed listening to Ben.

It was very enjoyable and during coffee afterwards Ben introduced me to Marion Studholme. She was as beautiful as she had been on the stage and had the bell-like speaking voice of a singer. During the conversation Ms Studholme asked Ben if she could see him afterwards and we ended up in our room which was a sort of study flat and quite presentable and comfortable. I joined them because I was so interested in talking to such a famous singer that I just tagged along without being asked and neither of them seemed to mind. After the usual scramble to find clean cups and make a brew, Ben's future began to shape before him.

Marion Studholme thought he had one of the best, young, baritone voices she had heard in recent years and quizzed him about his background. He had been a principal choir boy at Truro Public School gaining a scholarship there as a boy soprano. He had also sung as a boy on the radio. Ben explained that Cornwall, where he lived, had a very strong Methodist tradition and choirs were established all over the county. Singing in Cornwall was a tradition rather like the Welsh – probably the celtic influence beginning with blue woad and war chants!

After his voice broke at puberty, he had become too involved in school work and other things more exciting to a growing teenager, to think any more about singing. He was aware though, that he had a voice, which attracted attention even just when speaking and that people were always asking him to sing, especially in the pubs.

Marion Studholme then said "Have you ever thought about singing as a career and I'm talking about serious singing". Ben, of course, hadn't, which was why he was training to be a teacher. "Well, give the matter serious thought because I can introduce you to the Principal of the Guildhall College of Music and Drama here in London and, if he agrees with me, you could be offered a place there when you finish your studies here". She ended by giving him her telephone number.

The outcome was that she was true to her word. Ben was interviewed at the Guildhall, first by the Principal then by another person who was to become a great friend and influence on his life – Walther Greuner, a famous German singing coach who was a renouned expert on Lieder music.

For the rest of his time at Westminster Ben attended one afternoon per week at the Guildhall with Walter Greuner and then moved there as a full time student in 1959 after graduating from Westminster. While he was there, he became their most outstanding student winning the coveted Gold Medal before going on to greater things – Covent Garden, Glynebourne, Carnegie Hall and, of course, the "Geordie Proms". He was eventually awarded a fellowship of the college.

Well, Ben, I've written this about you because, try though I might, I have never been able to persuade you to write your autobiography as many of your contemporaries did. It is not your scene, "Mr Modesty", but if you had I know it would have been a good read depending on how many of your escapades you dared to tell. I am proud to have known you and I could not have asked for a more uplifting, rewarding and loving friendship, which has lasted between us for over 42 years now and I know this goes for Rosalynde too.

The tragedy in your life, which was to come, was serious deafness affecting both ears. This brought your great, international career to a premature end but not before the years of pleasure you gave to so many people on the operatic and concert stage, television and your many recordings. You have overcome this and bounced back, re-shaping your life in other ways but all, I'm delighted to say, linked to your love and feel for music. What better way to keep the Luxon name going than by producing operas and coaching budding singers. Even moreso is the fact that your daughter, Rachel, who has a beautiful soprano voice, is already following in your footsteps.

Chapter 6
My Career in Education and Raising a Family

I didn't teach in the classroom situation for very long. My first post was at Prudhoe County Secondary School and I sailed through my probationary year apart from shooting myself in the eye just before the school inspector came to see me teach. I think he got quite a shock when the Head said to him, "I'm sorry, Mr Walker has just shot himself in the eye and has been rushed to hospital". What a way to escape the dreaded inspector!

Actually, it wasn't as bad as it sounded but I had literally shot myself in the eye. It happened because I was teaching some Physical Education as well as Geography and I had gone into the P.E. Master's room to change. On his desk was a small automatic pistol, which I didn't recognise as a starting pistol. All the ones I had used had a cylinder barrel rather like a Colt 45. There was a water pistol craze going on at the school at the time and I thought my colleague had confiscated it from an unlucky pupil. I picked it up and without thinking pulled the trigger whilst looking down on the top of the gun not into the barrel. I received the full blast of cordite, or whatever it was, in both eyes. I thought I was blinded and sank down to the floor clutching my face in agony. Lorna Bell, the girls' P.E. Teacher, must have heard me scream from her changing room next door and came rushing in. Half an hour later, I was in hospital once again being treated for head injuries. They bathed both my eyes with a solution and bandaged me up so I couldn't see a thing. I stayed like that for several days until they removed the bandages and confirmed that my eyes had not received any permanent damage as the eyelids had taken the brunt of it – nature's protection at work. I was given drops to use for about a fortnight and gradually my sight returned to normal. It took a long time to live that incident down, especially in the staff room.

The rest of my probationary year passed uneventfully and I received a new class which was to stay with me for the next three years.

As a young, inexperienced teacher in the old secondary modern system you tended to be given classes of youngsters, who were not so academically inclined as their so-called brighter counterparts. Wrong really but that's another issue. I was very fortunate in that I was given a wonderful class of youngsters of quite varying ability, many of whom went on to further education and did very well.

I had one real challenge in this class and he was called Michael. He wasn't a nuisance or badly behaved, he just wasn't really interested in what I had to

28

say. I took them for most lessons and loved them all and will never forget them as my first class.

It was history one day and I was trying to interest them in Roman history, which abounds around the River Tyne near where I taught – the Roman Wall to the uninitiated. Try as I might I could not inspire any interest whatsoever in Michael so I had a word with the Head and he let me hire a bus. Later in the week, I took them all out to the Roman Wall for the afternoon also visiting one of the camps and its museum. They all seemed to enjoy it and I thought perhaps I was going to succeed at last as a teacher.

Before the next history lesson back at school, I prepared all sorts of visual aids etc for the blackboard and walls about the visit and looked forward to their reactions.

The lesson started something like this.......

"Well, everyone, I hope you all enjoyed your visit to the Roman Wall and before we start talking about what we've seen, has anyone anything they'd like to say about the trip?".

I said this with my eyes glued on Michael. He, for once, was sitting at a front desk where I could keep an eye on him, and, for once, was looking at me with more than an intelligent gleam in his eyes.

A number of hands short up and the usual chorus of "Sah! Sah! Sah!" (not sure how to spell this well heard classroom word) but miracles upon miracles, Michael's hand was up first!I pounced before it fell "Yes, Michael" I almost shouted in triumph. "Please, Sah!" he said "Your fly's open!!!" It was !

It was at Prudhoe that I became very interested in Youth Work. Northumberland Education Authority was pioneering the dual use of schools in the early sixties and they are now called Community Schools today. I became a voluntary Youth Leader at the School and started tennis and basketball coaching activities, which proved very popular. I became so interested in this type of work that I enrolled in the Authority's Introductory Training Courses for Youth Workers and eventually completed the Advanced Course. All of this took out great chunks of my personal time, which was already heavily committed to preparing lessons and marking books but I still managed to see Rosalynde mainly during weekends when I wasn't on training courses.

In 1961 we were married in an ancient Norman Church in Haltwhistle and we moved into a house in the village of Westerhope on the outskirts of Newcastle. It was a pretty house with a big garden and we still live there to this day. Rosalynde made great progress in her teaching career and successfully applied for the post of Head of Infants at a brand new Junior school, which was opened on the outskirts of the village.

In 1963 I applied for the post of Teacher Warden at Wideopen Secondary School and was successful too - our future in education looked secure. The post was to develop a youth association in the evenings and I was relieved of

One Lump or Two

Our Wedding Day on 12th August 1961

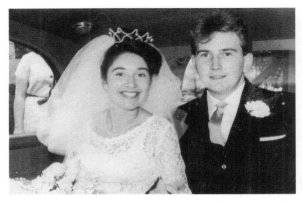

25% of my teaching time to work in the evenings. It was hard, back breaking work but I was paid a Deputy Head's salary, which wasn't bad for a 26 year old teacher. It wasn't like Prudhoe though where the Head and just about all the staff were dedicated to the Community School idea. I fought many battles with my new Head and staff but slowly, in time, I was able to convince them that their school would not be destroyed by the youth members and it would in fact benefit both the school and the neighbourhood.

The membership grew and grew and by 1967 I had one of the most thriving clubs in the county. Changes had just been implemented. The post of Teacher Warden disappeared as adult education moved in alongside the Youth Service. My new title became Further Education and Youth Service Officer and my teaching commitment was reduced to 50% during the day but my salary remained the same.

Rosalynde, too, was making great strides and was promoted to Deputy Head at her school at the very early age of 25. We were both very young to be in such senior positions, consequently we didn't see much of each other and we didn't lead a normal life. Things improved when Rosalynde joined me in my youth work and became a youth leader for me as well as running a thriving badminton group. We became a good team and the members responded to it.

This came to an end when we made one of the big decisions which face married couples - to have a family.

Before that, however, I cannot resist the opportunity to describe how my local reputation as a great lover was brought to everyone's attention and soared to heights to which even Casanova did not aspire. As a young couple carving out a career for themselves during these early years of marriage, we tried to be sensible about birth control and planned parenthood. We had spent our teens in the sedate 50s, which were then overtaken by the sexual revolution in the 60s and early 70s but I still found myself rather inhibited when it came to buying contraceptives at the local chemist shop.

This pressure was removed when a close friend told Rosalynde that contraceptives could now be obtained from the local health clinic at special monthly sessions and, better still, they were free! As this also took the onus

Marc & Roxanne in our back garden

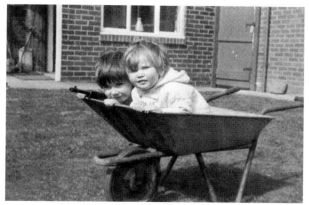

away from me because men didn't go to clinics in those days – male chauvinism or just simply scared, probably the latter – I persuaded Rosalynde to make the approach and I awaited her return with a mixture of trepidation and excitement – free contraceptives!

When Rosalynde returned she looked somewhat flustered and I was not sure whether the colour in her cheeks was due to fresh air or embarrassment. She plonked a small carrier bag on the table, which was bulging ominously, then tipped its contents out before sitting down. A large number of fair sized boxes tumbled onto the table and I picked one of them up. It read something like "Contraceptives – 1 dozen". There were 12 of these boxes. I looked quizzically at Rosalynde, who burst out laughing and said "I've never been so embarrassed in all my life" and proceeded to tell me what had happened.

First of all she said, "There's no real privacy, the nurse comes into the room, which was full of other women, presumably married, then proceeded to ask each of us what quantity we required. I was near the front of the queue and when it was my turn she asked me how many I wanted. As it was my first time I said I wasn't sure and so the nurse said it was usually a month's supply and asked me again how many I would need. I really didn't know what to say and I panicked after trying to make a hurried mental calculation so I blurted out that 12 would do.

The nurse gave me a funny look and turned to her cupboard behind her . I am sure the whole room went quiet, I didn't dare look around and waited for the nurse who turned and handed me these 12 boxes and a brown paper bag.

I mumbled my thanks and put the boxes into the bag and walked out of the room conscious that everyone was staring at me. When I got outside I checked the boxes and my reckoning is we've got 144 contraceptives to use before my next visit in 4 weeks time. No wonder everyone was staring at me. I asked for 12 contraceptives and she thought I meant 12 boxes. I'm not going back anymore, some of the women were mothers of the children I teach in school."

I couldn't help bursting out laughing at her predicament and for a long time afterwards I had the feeling that women were pointing me out in the streets whenever I went out shopping - a sort of local "superman", the Westerhope stud!!

Our son, Marc, was born on 23rd November, 1966 a beautiful baby with a thick mop of black hair. When we brought him home from the hospital and laid the carry cot on the kitchen table Rosalynde and I looked at each other helplessly and said,

"What do we do now?"

But we managed. Rosalynde resigned from her job and took on the more demanding role of wife and mother and I continued with my 40 sometimes 50 hour week in education.

I was rewarded for all this time and effort by beating all other applicants for the post of Deputy Headmaster (Further Education and Youth Service) at the Longbenton High School, which had the prestigious Robert Homes Youth and Adult Centre built on site at great expense only two years beforehand. I now had my very own premises, which included a Sports Hall, large canteen, dance hall and multi-purpose rooms. I had a full time Assistant Tutor and my own secretary. This was real promotion and a massive jump in salary.

I worked even harder those next few years and during that time our daughter, Roxanne, was born. She was a lovely, little blond-haired baby and the two of them were lucky to have the full time and energy of their devoted mother. I tried my best to be a good father but the job demanded much of my time and they often found me too tired to play with them or dashing out to work often at times that didn't suit them. The only consolation was that as I could take some time off during the day, I was able to spend time with them when other Dads were at work and when I went to work it was usually their bedtime. So there were "swings and roundabouts".

Roxanne was a good reader even from an early age and one night before I went off to work, I slipped up to her room to read her a story. She shared a room with Marc but he was allowed to stay up a little later. She was sitting up in bed, just bathed and looking very pretty. I sat on Marc's bed and opened her fairy story book. Appropriately, the story I chose was "Sleeping Beauty". After a few minutes the inevitable happened, it always did with me; I started to yawn and couldn't stop. It's rather like becoming sleepy when driving on the motorway. Roxanne came to my rescue this time and said, "Can I read, Daddy?", I gratefully handed her the book and stretched out on Marc's bed with my hands behind my head.

Next minute or so it seemed, I woke up with a start to find Rosalynde bending over me, shaking me and saying, "Wake up, it's 7.00 p.m. and you are late for work, what on earth have you been up to"? I sat up, Roxanne was still reading. I think she was on to her third or fourth story. I had fallen asleep for nearly three quarters of an hour. My staff didn't believe me when I got to work.

I remember a tutor on a training course telling me that she had left her husband looking after the children one day and came home to find him sitting in the play pen reading the newspaper while the children were running riot around the room.

In 1974 I was promoted into the job which I held for 4 years before making an unusual switch in 1978. The post was Education Adviser with the newly formed Metroplitan Borough of North Tyneside. There was a team of seven of us in those halcyon days of boundary re-organisation and a seemingly unending supply of money. There was one senior adviser and six advisers and our responsibility was the development of Adult Education and Youth Service throughout the borough. Looking back now, I can see that we were overstaffed but everything was new and exciting and perhaps we needed that size of team to get things off the ground. Four of the six were given area responsibilties and they moved out to offices on their own patch. Two including me, remained at headquarters, the Education Offices at North Shields, to work with the Senior Adviser and were given specific responsibilities. I think we were all carefully selected for the skills and experience we were best equipped to demonstrate. I had an overall brief for the school-based youth provision with special responsibility for developing and putting into practice a training scheme for all youth workers, most of whom were teachers. I became the Authority's officer responsible for the development and servicing of the Duke of Edinburgh's Award Scheme, which was really a voluntary thing but I was a great believer in it. Because of my great interest in outdoor education I was also responsible for the introduction and co-ordination of the youth service's use of 9 outdoor education centres, which were jointly shared and were run by the three North of the Tyne Authorities of Northumberland, Newcastle and my own new Authority of North Tyneside.

Exciting and challenging days and I threw myself into them with great enthusiasm. Much of the work was new to me. It was a great leap from running one's own centre in the sheltered, comfort of a school, to suddenly having borough-wide responsibility. I was now dealing with Headteachers, and Youth Officers on the same level. I was working alongside Directors of Education and all their Senior Staff, and also Councillors and Council procedure and they were all previously very dim and distant to me and now they suddenly played an important role in my work. They were our masters and providers of the money to enable us to do our job. It was a side of education that I vaguely knew existed but never dreamed I would ever work within their corridors of power.

Training of Youth Leaders, the Award Scheme and Outdoor education skills all had to take place at weekends and I had 30 weekends allocated to me on an annual basis from the Field Study Centre provision – a lot of weekends.

The centres were scattered around the wilder and most beautiful parts of Northumberland, with one exception, which was the Lake District near Windermere. Courses had to be planned well in advance advertised, costed and staffed and finally, members had to be transported there and back and this was only a small part of my job. They were, however, the times I enjoyed most because I was able to get back to the grass roots of the work I liked doing best, working with people and in particular young people. I am sure there are hundreds of people living now, who will look back with nostalgia on these centres, which gave them wonderful experiences of the real countryside and country life. Sadly, by the year 2000 there were only two of these centres left. The rest were the victims of drastic cuts in spending. They would be missed.

My two youngsters were growing up rapidly and Rosalynde had gone back to her old school to work. Not as Deputy Head this time but as Teacher in Charge of the newly established nursery school built on the site. We compensated for the many nights and weekends I had to work by the three of them coming with me on as many of the weekends as they could. This was only when there were spare places on the course. We also took every opportunity we could get to disappear together to our cottage in the Cheviots, which we bought in 1976 after having to relinquish the one we had rented since 1969.

During all this time my contact and awareness of ill health was limited to the children's illness and Rosalynde and I occasionally succumbing to colds and influenza viruses. I had been touched by cancer only really twice. The first was with Rosalynde's mother who died in 1962 without ever seeing her grandchildren or even knowing we would have them. This did not affect me as much as it perhaps should because this lady was a magnificent example of courage in the face of what was seen as a fatal illness in those days. Of all the years I knew her, I honestly never realised how seriously ill she was. She was always up and about and I never saw her without her looking her best, which must have needed great determination and strength of will. She and Rosalynde had a special relationship because Rosalynde had helped to look after her since she was 12 years old and I know she missed her mother terribly for many years after her death.

Cancer raised its ugly head close to me again when I was appointed to the post of Assistant Education Officer; a post which was split between Further Education, my forte, and Schools Education, which was new to me. It was an administrative post and I worked with the Assistant Director of Further Education and the Assistant Director for Schools. It was in the same Education offices but I was moved to the top floor, which in everyone's eyes was promotion indeed. I had made it and the world of education was my oyster! I knew everyone on the top floor of course but I was now one of them which seemed to make a difference. The only new man was Peter Brennan, who had only recently taken up the post of Assistant Director (Schools) coming from another Authority. He was a northeast man by birth and was really coming home to his roots. I worked closely with him for a while and was most impressed with his ability and humanity. He helped me over the many obstacles of my new post and I began to lose the doubts I had of whether I was capable of doing the job. I became very conscious of my academic inadequacies and struggled hard at keeping on top of things. The bewildering intricacies of the Education Act and the never-ending cycles of council minutes and meetings started to eat into my confidence. However, I struggled on and Peter and Harry Donkin, the other Assistant Director, who shared my services, were a great help to me.

It was then that tragedy struck and I saw for the first time how quickly cancer can attack and destroy. Peter Brennan confided in me one day that he had been experiencing severe headaches and a numbing sensation in his arm. Shortly after that he went on sick leave and the staff were shocked to hear that he had a brain tumour, which was inoperable. We all visited him at different times in the hospital where he had undergone surgery and was subsequently receiving radiotherapy treatment. I was dismayed at his appearance. One side of his head had been shaved and he had lost a lot of weight. He was still a young man with a very promising future ahead of him but here he was fighting for his life all in the space of a few weeks. I never thought he would come back to work but it was an indication of his fighting spirit when he did just that. Sadly, he was not the same man, he had been. His memory had been badly affected by the tumour or radiotherapy or both and it slowly drained his confidence. He battled on with great courage and was a hero in every sense. After a few months back at work he became ill again and on one very sad day, the Director informed us that he had died peacefully in hospital.

He was a Gateshead lad by birth and lived on that side of the River Tyne. The Church was packed with family and friends and colleagues from work on the day of his funeral. He would have been proud of his family that day, who fought back the tears to greet us all and particularly his eldest son, who stood up in front of the whole church and read a passage from the scriptures in a strong, clear voice, which only wavered slightly at the end.

His successor at work was another brilliant young man, Paul Eccles, who died under even more tragic circumstances a few years later. Suddenly life became more meaningful to me as I began to face the harsher realities of an existence, which hitherto had seemed secure and safe.

I worked with Paul for a short while until the retirement of two of the original six Further Education Advisers resulted in John Partington, the Director, reviewing the Service.

Mr Partington, or the "Boss" as he was affectionately called, invited me into his office one day and we talked for a long time about my future. He was a respected Director of Education and I always had a good relationship with him. His door was never closed to us and his advice carried me through many tricky problems, which came my way on the schools' side and needed more than my limited experience to handle.

He told me he had been pleased with my work as his Assistant Education

One Lump or Two

Officer but was aware that I was never happy being chained to a desk.

"I know you still get involved in the Award Scheme at weekends away with youngsters but really you should put that to one side if you want to make your career in Administration". I wasn't sure about that line of direction anymore and told him so.

"I need someone to go back into the field" were his next words, "with Sandy and Ernie retiring I cannot replace them because financial cuts are now beginning to bite. Jack Pentney has agreed to add Ernie's area to his but the problem area is Sandy's here in North Shields and Tynemouth. We must have someone in Sandy's Office to keep an eye on the Adult Education Centre, which as you know is the largest in the borough."

I knew that only too well as Sandy had let me establish a Duke of Edinburgh Award Centre and outdoor equipment store in a part of his huge building, which was standing empty. The Adult Centre had originally been the old Tynemouth Grammar School and was now shared with the newly built Tynemouth VI Form College, which was adjacent.

"You can remain as an Education Officer if you wish but your duties will obviously change and you may, if you wish, keep your training and Award Scheme responsibilities."

I didn't make my mind up immediately, the Director gave me time to think about it and talk to Rosalynde but like me, I think she knew where my heart lay.

I had six hard but fruitful and often enjoyable years at the Adult Education Centre. It was a house of many mansions, which included VI Form College use, Adult Education throughout the day and evenings and the thriving Duke of Edinburgh Award Centre. The Open University was based there as well as Adult Literacy. A later and most worthwhile addition became the teaching of life and social skills to mentally handicapped adults. They came on a day release basis from the borough's two Adult Training Centres. I even started a Special Star Award for them when they and the staff became interested in the Duke of Edinburgh Award Scheme. In 1980 when we were celebrating the 25th Anniversary of the Scheme. We had chosen to re-enact the "Song of the Lambton Worm" in front of the Duke at a grand, northeastern show staged especially for the anniversary at the Harrogate Showground. Meg Harrison, the teacher I had appointed to be in charge of the handicapped adults, was a great believer in their untapped skills. She was brilliant at bringing the best out of them and making them feel important to themselves and the community. With our help they built a magnificent "worm", which needed about 10 people inside to make it work and we transported it and its creators to the show and the combined groups put on a marvellous performance before Prince Philip and 5000 visitors.

At the beginning of 1987 this part of my life came to an end, more retirements and severe cuts in expenditure were making the Director pull in his belt several more notches. Harry Donkin was under great pressure; his advisory service was now down to one adviser, Jack Pentney, the last of the original magnificent seven, and the huge college of Further Education at Wallsend was taking up more and more of his time. Paul Eccles, the Assistant Director in charge of Schools was showing signs of the strain and needed a full time Assistant Education Officer.

The only way it could be done was for me to transfer back to an Educational Advisory post, enabling my post of Assistant Education Officer to attract someone with school's experience from another Authority. He knew I didn't want full time schools' work. My old office would be available to me back at the Education Offices. My assistant at the Adult Education centre would have to stand on his own two feet and run the place without my help. All part of the shrinking service!

And so I became a Senior Youth Adviser, this time with the overall responsiblity for the Youth and Community Service including the voluntary services and Jack Pentney was to take over the Adult Education service. Two of us were to do the work carried out by seven of us in 1974 because Harry Donkin himself retired a year after I returned to the Education Offices. This post was never filled up till the time I retired myself in September 1988 shortly after coming out of hospital having to face the most difficult battle of my life.

Prior to this it was becoming increasingly apparent that the years of continuous evening and weekend work, coupled with growing responsibility and additional workload, were beginning to take their toll on me. Stress, the hidden enemy which creeps up slowly but surely if there is no way to release it, finally revealed itself in different forms. Erratic sleeping patterns, bitchiness and quick temper, excessive coffee drinking, indigestion and I started smoking again - these were all symptoms I experienced.

A colleague once said to me

"You've stopped smiling and you don't make people laugh anymore". It was true and I hadn't realised it. Something had gone wrong and it certainly had as my first book "Cancer is only a Word" graphically describes the story and the outcome.

"Cancer is Only a Word" took up the story from there, which ended with our first North East Last Night of the Proms concert for Cancer Research and Patient Support on 20th October 1990.

Chapter 7
1994, St Paul's Cathedral & A Cricket Match

It seems very appropriate, having wandered briefly through my years before cancer, to pick up the threads where I left off in the epilogue of "Cancer is only a Word" in the summer of 1994.

It will help matters, however, if I briefly explain at this point of the story how the "North East Last Night of the Proms" was born as we then move into 1994 when the story really continues.

In 1988, the first lump appeared and was wrongly diagnosed as cancer of the pancreas and I was told I had about 12 weeks to live. The biopsy proved otherwise and I received a "reprieve". At the same time I set off on the long, very hard and very rocky road to fight and survive the cancer I was diagnosed with, Non-Hodgkins Lymphoma.

My treatment started in Spetember 1988 coinciding with Benjamin Luxon being chosen for the second time as the only baritone to sing Rule Brittannia etc. at the real Last Night of the Proms at the Royal Albert Hall - It was always a soprano before that.

Because of my predicament and Ben being Ben, he arranged for Rosalynde and I to be his guests and we enjoyed the most, wonderful musical evening of our lives. Our seats couldn't have been better - we were in a box next to Richard Baker, who was broadcasting the concert live on BBC Television.

A year later, wen I was recovering from an autologous bone marrow transplant, Rosalynde and I became aware that Steve Proctor was in danger of losing staff and beds which, in his line of business, meant that lives could be at risk.

Ben was visiting me at that time, taking a break from rehearsals at Covent Garden and I asked him if he would participate in a part fundraising concert and part "thank you for saving my life" concert for Steve's department. Ben immediately agreed and the discussion then evolved around what sort of concert, when and where.

To cut a long story short the idea of a "Geordie" Last Night of the Proms came up from Ben I think, and because of our experience in London, we thought it a wonderful idea. I managed to pin Ben down to a date, 20th October 1990 and a little later booked that date at the City Hall. So it all began in a semi-isolation room in Ward 8 at the RVI.

After that start we hadn't a clue where to go from there but, during that year, Rosalynde and I quickly learned the trade of concert production and ticket sales.

The result was a full house, Ben was brilliant, the evening was marred only by the fact that Janice Cairns could not appear with him because of a very unpleasant accident to her back, whilst performing Tosca at the Royal Coliseum in London.

At the end of the concert, a lady from the audience came onto the stage and made an impromptu speech on the audiences behalf and asked if they would like another "Geordie proms" next year ! We all looked at Ben aghast but he walked up to the microphone and said he'd enjoyed himself so much, he would be very happy to come back next year. The audience burst into ear-shattering applause and the North East "Geordie" Proms has never looked back since.

We were in the middle of preparation for the 5th "North East Last Night of the Proms" and needed a break. We had just spoken to Ben Luxon on the telephone about the programme and our pending visit to his farm in Kent and then on to attend another of his big concerts in London. The trip also included joining up with Janice Cairns, another famous singer who sang for us. She lived in Southampton with her husband, Mike, who was celebrating his 50th birthday with a cricket match followed by a party. We had all been invited and Ben and I were to play for his team after that we were to travel further afield again to stay with his mother in Cornwall where Ben was taking Master classes for budding opera stars. His London concert this time was to be held in St Paul's Cathedral. Ben had been invited by the Royal National Lifeboat Institute to sing Stanford's Songs of the Fleet. A very apt choice of music, which Ben had already recorded in 1983 with the Bournemouth Symphony Orchestra and Choir and which he had sung for us at our first concert in 1990. Wonderful, stirring music, which suited his voice to perfection.

It was another great occasion for us, which added more celebrity names to our list of people we had met through Ben. This time it was Timothy West and Patricia Routledge, who took turns in narrating the history of the Lifeboat Service through story and poetry interspersed with the music and songs by Stanford. Joanna Lumley was in the audience and we met her afterwards at a champagne supper held in the most macabre but fascinating place in which I've ever dined – the crypt of St Paul's Cathedral!

The food was excellent but I didn't really appreciate it as I was so intrigued by being literally surrounded by some of the most famous people in England's history. All dead, of course, but that only added to the excitement of the occasion.

Place of honour was given to Admiral Lord Horatio Nelson whose marble tomb was placed directly under the exact centre of St Paul's huge dome, which dominates central London. There was a small grille set in the floor directly above the tomb and when you look up you found yourself staring at the dome's centre spot.

The recent dead were honoured, too, as I found out when I stood in front of a large memorial to the Falklands War. There was a distinguished looking lady standing beside me and when I commented about the tragedy of it all, she said indeed it was and especially for her as she knew a number of naval personnel listed there. Intrigued by this, I asked her how that was so. She then introduced herself as Lady Fieldhouse and explained that her husband had been the Admiral in charge of the naval operations. I asked if he was with her that evening and felt rather embarrassed when she told me he had died recently; from natural causes not from anything sustained at the Falklands.

We proceeded to spend the next half hour chatting together. Ben was surrounded by admirers and Rosalynde was talking to Patricia Routledge so I was not being missed. Lady Fieldhouse was a very easy person to talk to, not what I expected from an Admiral's wife in the sense that, although we were poles apart in background, I felt very relaxed in her company probably because both our lives had been touched by tragedy.

She was intrigued that I had written a book and asked me to send her a copy when it was finally published and gave me her home address. We finally wandered over to Rosalynde who introduced us to Patricia Routledge. As my daughter, Roxanne, was a great fan of hers I told her that and then asked her if she would autograph my copy of the concert programme for her and took out my fountain pen.

"I don't sign autographs on occasions like this", she said in a rather off hand manner, which left me quite taken aback and embarrassed. I could see Rosalynde was embarrassed for me too so I just mumbled something in reply. Lady Fieldhouse took me by the arm and led me off to her table, skilfully changing the subject and sparing me any further embarrassment. Rosalynde followed almost immediately and the three of us enjoyed the rest of the evening together until, eventually, Ben and Sheila managed to drag themselves away from the organisers.

After prolonged farewells we set off on the long journey back to Kent. I've never liked the comedy programme "Keeping up Appearances" or the character of Mrs Bouquet but liked both even less after that encounter. Much later I remembered to send Lady Fieldhouse a copy of my book and received a very nice letter and donation in reply.

We spent the next few days in glorious sunshine helping Ben tidy up his vegetable garden, cutting the grass and swimming, sunbathing and barbequing around his pool. Finally we set off for Southampton for Mike's 50th birthday party and the cricket match.

Mike is a professor of oceanography at Southampton University and an avid cricketer. He and Janice met on a train travelling to London where she is a principal singer for English National Opera and Janice told me that as soon as she saw him she decided he was the man she was going to marry. Only a Northumbrian lassie can be as decisive about her man as that! Janice was born in Ashington, Northumberland. Rosalynde and I were both touched that we'd been invited to the celebration and although I haven't played cricket since school days I was looking forward to the match and meeting their family.

It turned out to be great fun. Ben and I played for Mike's team against a team from the University captained by a friend and colleague of Mike. I had borrowed some whites and wore my white golfing shoes. Ben was resplendent in a Victorian striped blazer, cap and white flannels, which he wore in the Covent Garden production of "Die Fledermaus", which I have mentioned in an earlier chapter. They had been given to him as a momento and were ideal for the day.

Mike's team took the honours, he himself batting undefeated to the end. I scored 12 runs and took three wickets. Ben was bowled out first ball but as the rule that day did not permit that, he continued batting for a further three balls before being bowled out for the second time. Nevertheless, he was definitely the smartest player on the field! After tea in the pavilion, the hired bus returned us to Janice's house but not before stopping at the pub on the way to celebrate or commiserate depending on which team you represented. There I found myself chatting to Janice's family and close relatives from Ashington. After over a week in the South of England, it was heart-warming to be surrounded by people speaking with the soft burr of Northumberland and we got along like a house on fire. Although the conversation was mainly about the match it inevitably drifted to our concert in Newcastle. They had all been to the previous ones because of Janice's involvement and were full of praise for our efforts, and were all going to the next one in October.

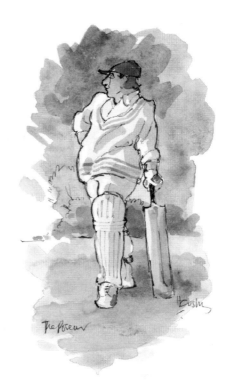

Back at Janice's home, a marquee had been erected in the back garden where the celebrations continued well into the night. There were a few sore heads in the morning including my own but it had been a wonderful day helped even more by fine sunny weather.

Next day, after fond farewells with Janice and Mike, we set off for Cornwall visiting Winchester Cathedral on the way.

The "poseur" - who, Mike, Ben or George?

41

Chapter 8
A Meeting with a Mezzo Soprano

Cornwall is a beautiful county with the added benefit of warmer climes than our part of the country but this has its drawbacks in the huge number of holidaymakers, who descend on the place every summer.

Fortunately Ben's mother's house is slightly off the beaten track near a small village called Goldsitheny. It lies midway between the narrow neck of Cornwall so you have the choice of two coastlines a few miles in opposite directions. We tended to go to the north side where it was quieter and wilder with exciting cliff walks looking down on sandy bays. Ben had bought the house for his mother, Lucille, and step-father, Jack, years earlier and we have all spent many happy holidays with them as our respective children grew up.

Jack's surname was Cock, which must have taken some living with and I remember when my son, Marc, was only about four or five years old and we were staying with Lucille and Jack along with Ben, Sheila and their family. Marc became a Cornish pastie addict and was immensely impressed by Lucille's preparation and cooking of them. When we were on the beach one day and the children were playing on the sand and I went for a swim. Suddenly a very big fish swam close to me and proceeded to drift towards the beach. I left the water very slowly so as not to disturb it and picked Marc up to show him. As we entered the water it turned and swam out to sea but Marc caught a brief glimpse of it.

Marc was very excited by it and said we should have caught it. He then uttered his first very amusing "spoonerism".

"What a pity, daddy, it got away, we could have taken it home and Mrs Cook could have cocked it up for us!"

For Ben this was a working holiday. He was giving three days of Master Classes for singers at Lanhydrock – a beautiful stately home, which had been taken over by the National Trust, and after that he was taking part in a national network of music scheduled to go out all over the British Isles from various points along the coastline: Ben along with the Marazion Male Voice Choir was representing Cornwall and the broadcast was from Lands End cliff tops.

Lanhydrock was first, however, and we were to be part of the audience. Ben's daughter, Rachel, had discovered she had a gifted soprano voice like her mother and had decided to make singing her career. She travelled down with us and was taking part as a pupil. As I listened to her perform before her father I realised that she had a beautiful voice and I couldn't help wondering if she would ever follow in her parent's steps and sing for us one day in the City Hall at Newcastle – a thought which would eventually become a reality but that was way into the future.

Before that event was to take place something else happened during those

Master Classes, which had a profound affect on our North East Last Night of the Proms and this led to the formation of another annual concert, which became a very popular event with our supporters.

When Ben was staying with us up North, he would often talk about Cornwall and two things in particular. One was his dream of a concert hall for Cornwall and he was President of a county-wide campaign for it and the other was his involvement with Duchy Opera – an amateur company based in Truro of which he was patron. He also made guest appearances in their annual opera performances and coached some of their principal singers when he had the time available. One singer in particular was a farmer's wife who, according to Ben, was not only a beautiful, striking young woman but had a wonderful voice too. He said she had the potential to become a star in her own right if she wanted to but it would involve a substantial sacrifice as she had two young children and helped her husband, William, to run a large dairy farm near St Austell.

During the master classes, each singer performed prepared pieces and Ben helped them in the way only he can do, always enthusiastic and always encouraging. He deftly slipped in improvements to their voice, posture, their understanding of the music without belittling their ability or embarrassing them in any way. He was a natural teacher and brought out the best in every performer.

There were a variety of voices and a variety of songs, which never permitted the day to become boring but two voices, in particular, stood out for me. Firstly, of course, was Ben's daughter, Rachel, who sang really well and the other Ben simply introduced as Suzanne and everyone seemed to know her. She sang like an angel and she oozed sex appeal, in the nicest possible way. When she had finished Ben simply said, "Suzanne, that was first class, there is nothing I can say or add to your performance, well done".

The name suddenly clicked, I looked at my list of singers and saw the name Suzanne Manuell, Manor Farm, St Austell. So this was the woman that Ben kept mentioning and I could see why – but she looked much younger than I expected – a mere lassie rather than a farmer's wife with two children and what a voice!

I immediately thought "I have to have her!" and, before anyone jumps to conclusions, I meant to perform in Newcastle at our Last Night. At that point Ben said "I know you have to dash now to pick up the children from school but I look forward to seeing you again later in the year at Duchy Opera's next production".

Suzanne smiled in acknowledgement and slipped out of the room. As this was the last day of the classes, I knew I only had one opportunity to make contact with Suzanne and that had to be before she reached her car. To Rosalynde's surprise I jumped to my feet and hurried out of the room after her.

Fortunately, it was a long walk down the front driveway to the car park and I managed to catch up with Suzanne in time. Coming up behind her I called out her name and she stopped, turned and looked at me somewhat surprised.

"I'm George, Ben's friend from Newcastle" I blurted out not knowing what else to say in the way of introduction.

Obviously Ben must have mentioned me to her because she said she knew who I was. I then said how much I'd enjoyed hearing her sing and explained about our concert. I could see she was wondering what it was all leading up to so I got to the point and asked if she would like to sing for us in Newcastle. Her reaction was an immediate yes. Knowing she was in a hurry I said I'd be in touch with her through Ben and quickly explained it would not be this year's concert as the programme was already more or less arranged. So we parted and the seeds were sewn. October 1995 seemed a long way off but the contact had been made.

It was at the 1994 concert that we introduced another "Cornishman", by adoption not by birth; his name was Derrick Phoenix with a wonderful tenor voice. He was a bank manager in Truro and he met Ben by accident at the bank. He recognised Ben, of course, and talked at length with him about his love of singing. This was the beginning of a long friendship welded even closer when Ben discovered Derrick had indeed an excellent singing voice, which led him into many leading roles in operas produced by the Cornish company, Duchy Opera, of which Ben was President. It naturally followed that when we told Ben we thought it was time we had a tenor to widen the variety of arias and songs, Derrick became our man. He received a great welcome from our audience at his debut and continued to sing as one of the "team" until his untimely death from a heart attack in the summer of 1998 but that is into the future.

It was several months later before I was able to confirm with Suzanne that she had a part to play and I was impressed by her enthusiasm and eagerness to join us. Her farm was about 580 miles from Newcastle, a round trip of over 1000 miles, a long way to travel for a couple of hours on the stage at the City Hall but the "Geordie audience" loved her when she finally made it. When people found out she was from Cornwall they began jokingly describing it as a Cornish takeover.

Before we returned North we drove to Lands End with the Luxon family and joined the crowd on a cold, wind-swept cliff watching Ben and the choir perform "And Shall Trelawney die" over the country's network radio linking up with other areas for National Music Day. The song is not a favourite with Ben and he revised it en route. He got his words mixed up during the broadcast but

I don't think anyone noticed, they were so busy trying to keep warm. There was an Irish folk singer there to who sang a lovely folk song. I recognised him as Noel Murphy who made the very amusing song "Murphy's Bricks" very popular in the 1970s. Years later in the new Century 2001 I met him again at a Golf Club in Cornwall when Rosalynde and I were playing golf with Dr Anthony Seddon, Suzanne's accompanist, and his friend. We had drinks together in the clubhouse, where he was a member, having settled nearby in one of the lovely Cornish fishing villages. We all bought a CD of his favourite songs from him which included "Murphy's Bricks" and which he just happened to have in his locker in the changing room!

All good things come to an end and back home, we started preparation to drastically modernise our cottage in the Cheviots as well as sort out work for the concert which was rapidly looming on the horizon.

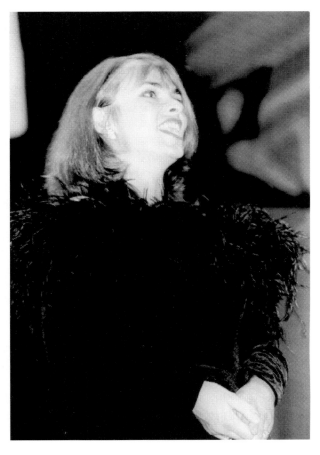

Suzanne Manuell - her first appearance at the "Geordie" Proms, 1996

Chapter 9
Another Lump & Demolition Time

Duringall this time and all these events I haven't mentioned cancer. It isn't because it wasn't there, it was but life was so full that I could keep it in the background most of the time.

At the 1993 concert I had announced to the audience that I had just completed my first tumour-free year. Uplifting words but I had spoken too soon and in December of that year a small lump appeared under my arm. Steve Proctor had examined it but thought it was a normally occurring lymph node and decided to just keep an eye on it.

I hoped he was right but deep down I wasn't that confident and continued my own regular checks of all the likely places where a lump could appear. This is a nerve racking experience in itself and I always heave a sigh of relief when nothing is found. The small lump under my arm didn't change, however, and I had to be careful not to probe there too firmly as it could become sore from the pressure and that could add more fear as the imagination responded.

My record so far in "lump" statistics was:- the big one in 1988, one in the groin in 1990, two more in the kidney area in 1991, my neck in 1992 and later that year I found one under my arm whilst on holiday in Israel. Then came the "lump-free" year until the present one appeared under my arm. So far I had received chemotherapy, an autologous bone marrow transplant, surgery, intensive radiotherapy, more chemotherapy and then a further dosage of radiotherapy. It is truly amazing how much punishment the body can take, still continue to function normally and then recover. My hopes of winning took a huge knock with each occurrence and this required a mental recovery every time, too, which was just as difficult and energy sapping as the physical recovery.

My physical recovery is helped considerably with my enjoyment of exercise in the form of golf, tennis, cycling, walking in the Cheviots, yoga and gardening. Not in any particular order but I'm really enjoying my golf at the moment. My mental recovery is helped by keeping busy and running a registered charity with Rosalynde from our home. This provides many challenges but there is a lot more to it than that.

You can never underestimate the power of love, which comes at me from all sides. From Rosalynde, Roxanne and Marc, my close friends and neighbours to the many people I have come to know through our concerts and my book. My medical friends play their part too in this form of therapy. They are always there for me, as they are with their other patients, with immediate back up when things go wrong and always a smile plus words of encouragement when they are most needed. But it still comes down to yourself in the end, especially during the moments when you find yourself alone or the fear becomes so great that there is the temptation to shrink into a corner, cover your head with your hands and cut yourself off from reality. It is at this time you have to call upon your own reserves of strength to shake off the fear and find something, no matter how small, to remind you that you've got to keep fighting.

This has happened to me several times and the usual cause is finding another lump or some unexplained symptom, which leads to the conclusion, which is more often than not wrong, that the cancer is back. When this happens my first reaction is always to keep it to myself. I do this because my assumptions may be wrong and I don't wish to worry any one else unnecessarily. This may last for quite some time until I am reassured or I am convinced something is terribly wrong. I then need help and, of course, the first person I turn to is Rosalynde and then Steve Proctor. Rosalynde does not agree with this approach. She quite rightly accuses me of cutting myself off from her and our family and friends. My usual answer to this, which is not a fair one, is to say "Swap places with me for a short while and then tell me what you would do". It is very difficult for people, who have never experienced a life threatening illness or have never gone through very unpleasant but, no other choice treatment, to understand. It is also very difficult for people with life threatening illnesses to understand the equally traumatic feelings their loved ones have to cope with and for just as long. In my last book I stressed bringing cancer out into the open, even the title was a message about it but at certain times it is easier said than done. My illness, as I once said at a fundraising banquet, has become a very public one. At this particular banquet, which Rosalynde had organised, I was in the middle of more chemotherapy; a stronger dose than usual because the tumour which had appeared was a rather nasty one and had to be hit hard. I had lost my hair again and weight. I did not want to go to the banquet because I would have to face about 150 people, most of whom thought I was fit and well. Cancer treatment does not always leave you to appear looking normal and there was no way I could escape this particular confrontation. I expressed my fears to Rosalynde, who sympathised but reminded me that this is what our work was all about and, if everything else I had done since 1988 meant anything, I had to face everyone. She was right, of course, and I went. I even stood up and spoke to everyone making a joke about the situation in my usual style.

There was a spontaneous outburst of clapping when I finished and after that the evening went better for me than I expected and was to help me through other public confrontations in the weeks that lay ahead. However, that is further into the future and I still had another lump to contend with first.

My misgiving mentioned at the beginning of this chapter became fact when I found a similar small lump in my neck. This time it was above the right collar bone – the nine months wait was over and for the worst possible reasons. I visited Steve before I told Rosalynde, which was out of character but I was hoping I might be wrong and wouldn't have to disappoint her too. Steve confirmed it but reassured me that it was low grade and felt that a small dose of radiotherapy would do the trick and that I could have the lump under my arm treated in the same way and at the same time. He said he would make the necessary arrangements with Helen Lucraft, the Consultant Clinical Oncologist and Radiologist, at the Newcastle General Hospital, who had treated me successfully on more than one occasion.

In the meantime Rosalynde and I became heavily involved in major alterations to our cottage as well as coping with concert ticket sales and preparing for a September holiday to Canada for three weeks with the Goodarzi family. Margaret Goodarzi had been a pupil of mine at Wideopen Secondary School, worked for me later as a Youth Leader, was our first babysitter and married an Iranian friend called Fari, who gained his PhD in Petrology at Newcastle University. They became our neighbours for a short while before settling in Canada where Fari is a Professor at Calgary University. They have a son and two daughters and we were looking forward to seeing them all again, but I'm digressing...............

Our cottage at Kypie Hill Farm on the eastern edge of the Cheviots has played a major part in helping me through the early days of my treatment offering me peace and quiet, fresh, clean air, wonderful views, very friendly people and access to the Cheviots and the golf course at the Hirsel, Coldstream. We had sunk all our saving into it in 1976 and since then had spent as much time there as we could.

Although we had already done a lot of restoration work to it especially to the gardens, we finally decided to make it easier to live in and more comfortable and cosy. It was a big decision and started with a complete rewiring of all the electrics. We were lucky that a neighbouring farmer and friend, Ian Ainsley, had served his time as an electrician whilst his parents ran the farm. As the farm became bigger, Ian joined his parents and only did occasional electrical work when time permitted. He made an excellent job of the cottage including putting in night storage heaters where they were needed although we kept the original open fire and stove which heated the water and cooked mouth-watering casseroles while we were out walking. We had already installed secondary glazing, keeping the original

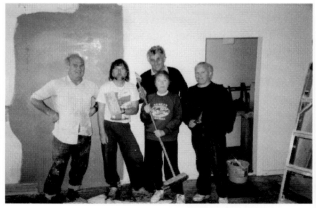

The "demolition" team at the cottage

48

windows, so the place was now going to be much warmer especially in the cold, windy days of winter.

The job we were about to begin was knocking out the very tiny kitchen and the larder, which was actually bigger than the kitchen and turning the area of the larder and the small downstairs bedroom into a more spacious kitchen and dining room. The original kitchen, which was actually in the lounge area would make the living room into a much bigger room and add an extra window and viewpoint of the garden to it. We had planned a "demolition" weekend bringing up our friends, John and Eileen Thompson and Alan and Margaret Young, under the "supervision", for want of a better word, of Andy Spears, who had helped us with the original restoration work. Andy was the "gourmet" of the building world. You name it he could do it, he was brilliant and a lovely chap at the same time.

We all bedded down at our cottage and Emily, our next door neighbour, loaned us the use of her cottage and we worked non-stop over the weekend. Fortunately it was sunny and all our downstairs furniture was moved outside before the demolition began. By the end, it looked like a bombsite but the major work was done. During the following week Ian, the electrician, moved in with his plasterer friend and when we returned the next weekend, we reassembled the kitchen, replaced the furniture, which had just been dumped indoors and started decorating. The dust was the worst problem but we eventually won the battle and by the third weekend things were back to normal. We all celebrated with a meal at the Blue Bell pub down the road near Crookham.

Since then we have had the place carpetted, Alan and I laid sandstone flags in the kitchen area and we bought a new and very comfortable four piece suite which complemented the new, large lounge.

All this hectic activity kept my mind off those two lumps and became a therapy in itself. Eventually, I had to face them and soon after completion of the work I received an appointment with Dr Lucraft at Newcastle General Hospital where it had all began in 1988. This time it was quick and painless. Helen worked out the doseages for each lump based on the information which Steve Proctor sent to her. She checked the lumps herself, of course, and seemed satisfied. I received one treatment on each of the small lumps – about two minutes per lump, I think – and that was that. She assured me they would disappear in a few weeks time and they did, to my great relief. Another battle over and probably the quickest, cleanest victory I had had up till then.

The lump under my arm disappeared first; the one in my neck took a little longer. It disappeared, in fact, during our Canadian holiday in September – no one knew about it except Rosalynde and my doctor friends. Consequently I was able to enjoy Calgary, Edmunton and long trips into the Rocky Mountains, staying at Jasper and Banff sleeping over in log cabins with the Goodarzi family. We had a wonderful time with them and we are determined to visit them again sometime in the future, if all is well.

Chapter 10
A Break from Writing

This next chapter is an escape from cancer, hospitals, concerts and fundraising.

I'm taking a break at our cottage to continue my story but, just as in the first book, I took its readers on a couple of my walks in the Cheviots as a form of escapism, I'm about to do the same again.

I've been writing away steadily for two days and have a strong urge to stretch my legs and breathe some fresh country air. As I look up from this manuscript I stare at an oil painting I bought in Coldstream whilst shopping for food. It was a spontaneous decision but I've learned from bitter experience in the collecting "game" that you should buy it if you like it. If you leave it to another day you can be sure it will have gone – bought by another collector or dealer who has learnt how to make up his or her mind at once. This time I had and Rosalynde hasn't the slightest idea what I've done as she is back home in Newcastle. It's an oil painting of a beautiful young girl who looks as though she has just let her hair down. She is looking very wistful and I've spent lengthy moments wondering what was going through her mind. I have no idea who the artist is but it is late Victorian or certainly very early 20th century and well painted. The girl reminds me very much of Rosalynde when she was a teenager and I'm hoping that romantic notion will help her to accept why I've bought yet another painting in my 30 years of collecting. Rosalynde gets a "bee in her bonnet" about my "collectophobia" and it is not just paintings. I've been a collector all my life from geological and fossil specimens to woodcarvings, antique plates to furniture, and paintings to old brass bells. Paintings are my real love, however, and I never tire of looking at my collection. It is not a valuable one but I always get a terrific buzz when I find a painting, which hasn't already been discovered by another collector.

I tore myself away from the painting before I could start dwelling on the reception the painting and I would receive when Rosalynde saw it. Then after dressing myself for the outdoors, I built the fire up, placed the guard in front of it and stepped out into the cold, bracing air. Once outside, I decided to have a long walk. It is a Sunday and I thought I'd set off early and walk over to and around Ford Moss, timing it to have Sunday lunch at the Red Lion in Milfield – it is always an excellent lunch and very reasonable. It was cold and grey when I set off with spots of rain in the air but it was invigorating and just what I needed.

Ford Moss is about six miles from the cottage and is an ancient bog, which had formed over hundreds of years consisting of accumulated vegetation filling up a natural basin with a high water table, which prevents vegetation from rotting. There are not many natural bogs left in this country for all sorts of reasons and most of them due to man's relentless destruction of the countryside. This particular one belongs to the estate of Lord Joicey of Etal Manor but it has come under the care of the Northumberland Wildlife Trust – an organisation dedicated to the preservation of the natural countryside.

To reach it I had to skirt a large heather and bracken covered hill called Goatscrag Hill via Routing Linn, a small but impressive waterfall hidden in a wooded valley near the hill. Nearby there are some fine examples of "cups and rings" as they are called. They are ancient carvings on small rock outcrops and they can be found in a number of places in North Northumberland. No one really knows their origin or significance but many believe they are linked to sacrificial rituals well before Christianity was born.

I couldn't pass without seeing the waterfall and the carvings again and as I detoured I met another lone walker, the only one I'd seen for the last hour. He turned out to be an ornithologist "policing his beat" for bird surveying statistics and we had a long and interesting chat. Apparently experienced members of the Northumberland Bird Society are given set areas to cover throughout the year. Their job is to record bird sightings at given times within their designated area. This helps the Society to keep track of bird movements, population density and how they are affected by weather, scarcity of food, pollution and so on. While we were talking he said "That was a meadow pipit over there". I hadn't heard or seen anything but having been out several times with Rosalynde's cousin-in-law, who is an expert bird-watcher, I wasn't surprised. The real experts can spot or hear a bird and identify it before the keen but inexperienced enthusiast has even thought of raising his binoculars.

I left him to his work and continued on my way. The waterfall was quite a sight after weeks of continuous rainfall and the cups and rings, in their protected, fenced area; never fail to make me ponder about the mysteries of life. I stared at them in the way I usually do trying to picture early man working on them and for what reason – a reason we'll never know.

I then headed for Southmoor Farm before swinging southwest to Dovehill Crag, which looms over Ford Moss. The fields I crossed were wet and boggy from all the recent rain even before I reached the Moss so I wondered how safe the bog was. I couldn't walk on it anyway as it is now fenced off and only the Society's members are permitted access to it. It is, however, clearly visible and there is a display board covered with interesting information about the bog and its habitat. As I approached this I passed a ruined stone building, which still had signs of industrial usage inside it, as though an engine of some sort had been installed there. Nearby were a number of small rectangular-shaped fences. I remembered that these were covering the sites of bell pits, a very early method of extracting coal, which was found near the surface. The coal miners dug deep, bell-shaped holes in the ground and carried the coal out by means of

Looking from Ford Moss towards the Cheviots

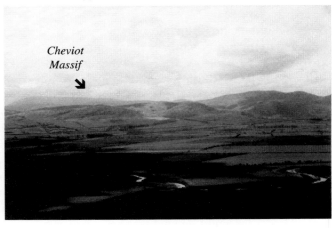

Cheviot Massif

ladders. When they had dug as deeply as they could safely manage they then simply dug another pit and so on. The holes were now filled in and protected by the fences. Nearby were the remains of the miners' rude homes where they lived and eked out a pretty miserable existence.

The last thing I saw as I left the bog was the tall chimney built on a small outcrop at the edge of the moss. This chimney was all that was left of the pump house, which had pumped water out of the mine workings and eventually took over from the bell pits. It now stood as a monument to a nearly forgotten age – a small industrial island surrounded by thousands of acres of farmland. Far away in the distance I could see the 'Cheviot Massif, which was covered in cloud at the top but there was enough light to highlight the lower slopes and surrounding hills and for all the bleakness of a grey Northern day, there was still a feeling of wonder and majesty about the scene. I just stared at it for a long time; soaking up the strength these hills always seemed to give me.

It was a gentle downhill walk all the way to the Red Lion after that and an hour later found me in the lounge sitting beside a glowing wood stove, a pint on the table and chatting to Malcolm, the landlord. Rebecca Craig, the daughter of the local doctor, who sold me delicious free range eggs whenever I called, was also there along with Malcolm's mother and step-father, who were visiting. They all go to our Last Night of the Proms (a 100 mile round trip) so the conversation inevitably centred on that and our plans for the next one.

After a delicious Sunday lunch and some sparkling conversation, I reluctantly dragged myself away from the cosy warmth of the pub and set off back to the cottage. It was raining by then and the last couple of miles were not as enjoyable as the rest but it was still a walk I would recommend to anyone. For me it had been a pleasant interlude and I was in a much more relaxed mood by the time I stirred the fire, switched on some music and settled down to continue this story.

Chapter 11
France, Norway and Yet Another Lump!

1995 was a strange mixture of events including a combination of three weeks away skiing and a fantastic trip to America culminating on Martha's Vineyard – holiday island of the rich!

The first trip was to Valloire in France looking after the Newcastle General Hospital Ski Club, many of whom were now very close friends of mine having taught quite a few of them to ski since I first joined them in 1989. The snow was good and this time my son, Marc, joined us. It was the first time I'd skied with him for a number of years, due to college studies and other challenges in his life. He hadn't lost his touch and by the end of the first day I had a difficult job to keep up with him. Everyone in the group commented on what an excellent skier he was, not surprisingly since he was only five years old when I first put him on skis, which he took to like a duck to water. We had a great week which was heightened for me by the chance for father and son to share a common bond.

Poor Rosalynde had fared less well. She had been invited by a close friend and neighbour, Kath Baker, who owned a flat with her husband in Flaine, another top ski resort in France. It was to be a "girls week", which was marred by really poor weather conditions. While we enjoyed snow and sunshine in one resort she had to put up with rain, wind and slush in another. It was so bad she even managed a refund on her lift pass, which is quite an achievement from the French!

My second trip was as ski party leader in charge of a party of teachers and pupils from two different local schools visiting the Voss ski resort in Norway. There were about 72 of us altogether and snow conditions were very good. It was very hard work but the staff and youngsters were a pleasure to work with and we all had a wonderful time together. When we set off from Newcastle Airport, I could tell everyone was weighing me up and wondering what sort of leader they had been landed with but something happened on the journey, which broke the ice and the rest of the week took off from there.

While everyone was waiting for their baggage to be loaded from the plane on to the buses in Norway, one of the Air Stewards from the flight asked me if I'd follow her back to the plane. Apparently a ventolin inhaler and some tablets had been found on the plane. It took about 25 minutes to sort that out and when I returned to the terminal there was no sign of the half a dozen teachers and 70 children. I stood looking around me rather puzzled because the teachers knew I'd gone back to the plane. I rushed outside where the buses had been waiting but there was no sign of them anywhere. My skis and boot bag and other luggage had vanished too! Within minutes of landing in Norway, the party leader had lost his party!

I dashed back into the terminal and found an official, who could help me; fortunately most Norwegians speak English. He sensibly contacted the bus company, the name was on my documents and they were able to contact the buses by radiophone. They were just leaving the city and one turned back while the other pulled into a lay-by and waited.

The teachers were very embarrassed, each bus thought I was on the other and in the scramble to load and leave they had forgotten I had to return to the plane. I couldn't help wondering whether I was going to be obsolete to the trip but as events turned out I was able to give them all a week, which everyone enjoyed, without any real problems or disasters and improve their skiing at the same time. The letters I received from everyone afterwards made up for the hard work and long hours, which are very necessary when looking after a large group of young people in a foreign country. Regardless of the glamour, skiing is still a dangerous sport.

The third trip was to Cesano, which was on the border between France and Italy. This was with the hospital group again but I was on holiday and this time Rosalynde was with me. This resort is linked to Sestriere, Sauze D'ouix and Montegenevre so we had four resorts to ski. It was towards the end of the season and the weather was good, too good at times because the snow melts and then becomes icy, making skiing difficult. However, we skied all the resorts and had a super week, during which I also experienced one of those rare moments of life through racing ahead of the group I was leading, to stop the lift going down to Cesano from closing and leaving us stranded. I sped round a bend on the piste cutting steeply down a wooded slope to be confronted by a magnificent stag standing in the middle of the piste with three female deer beside him. He had a wonderful spread of antlers and he just stood there like a king, lord and master of all around him. I skidded to a halt just feet from them and covered them in a spray of snow and we just stared at each other, all in shock. I hoped the rest of the group would catch me up to witness this moment but with a toss of its head, the stag turned, and followed by the hinds, disappeared into the wood. An unforgettable moment.

Did anything occur to spoil all this physical winter enjoyment? Sadly, yes. In Norway, whilst showering at the end of a hard day's skiing, I felt an uncomfortable feeling in my groin and automatically probed the area with my fingers. I wish I hadn't but it was too late, I had found another lump. No amount of probing could make it disappear and I just had to get on with the rest of the week until I returned home and had it checked out.

For once, and this is the only time this has happened in almost 14 years, the lump did not turn out to be a tumour. I went through all the usual procedures and had to, once again, contend with my fears and disappointment. I told Rosalynde as soon as I returned home. I hate doing this because I see the pain

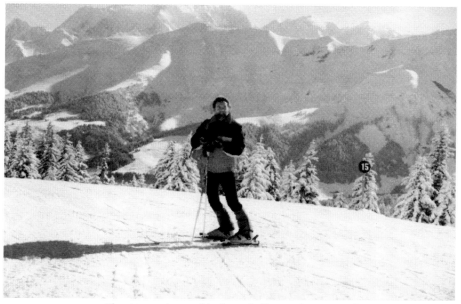

About to go down a black run in France (very steep!)

and sympathy for me in her eyes every time I have to put her through it and, just like me, I know she has to steel herself for what could be ahead.

I received a very quick appointment with Steve Proctor, who examined me, concentrating on the groin area. "Cough for me, George, please" which I did with a resurging memory of my National Service medical years ago. "You have a hernia" said Steve, after I had to cough another couple of times, "this is not a lymph node". What a relief! I felt the gloom and doom lift from my shoulders and couldn't wait to return home and tell Rosalynde the good news. The irony of all this is that I was now faced with a painful operation and fairly long recovery period; longer for me because I had such a physically active life, but I am describing it as "good news"! Several weeks later I went through the operation and slowly recovered. Life returned to normal or as normal as my life can be.

I made a meal of it in my speech on stage at the next Last Night of the Proms in the following October. Each year I gave a humorous bulletin about my progress to the audience and this always includes a joke or two about Steve Proctor and the medical world. This year was no exception and the audience laughed with me as I spouted forth.

Chapter 12
Trip to America and Martha's Vineyard

Our trip to America took place before that particular "Prom"and it was another great highlight for us.

It all came about because of Ben. He had been flying to Boston in the early 80s to sing at Tanglewood, home of the Boston Symphony Orchestra. The flight was diverted because of fog and he shared a room with a man he had met on the plane before completing the journey. Jim Barrett, a Consultant Psychiatrist, turned out to be a fan of his and they became great friends. Another of Jim's friends, Bob Blacklow, who was Dean of Medicine at Ohio University, joined that friendship and Ben stayed with them after that every time he performed in their respective parts of America. I mentioned Bob Blacklow briefly in my first book when he attended the 1988 Last Night of the Proms as a guest of Ben. He joined us in the box next to Richard Baker, who was broadcasting the concert live for BBC Television.

Between them they had persuaded Ben and Sheila to come over to America on a sort of working holiday. Ben was to give master classes to budding opera singers at Hanover University and the arrangement was for Jim and them to join Bob and his wife, Wini, at their holiday home on Martha's Vineyard to give a concert with Sheila to the islanders. They accepted and Bob, who had met Rosalynde and me at the London Proms, invited us to join them on the island. Jim Barrett and his English wife, Jane, without knowing us, asked us to join them in Hanover where they had arranged the master classes for Ben. So we experienced America for the first time.

Where were our experiences through cancer going to end?

We spent two weeks in Hanover, New England, then two weeks at Martha's Vineyard. New England is the largest forested, area in the whole of America. Jim and Jane lived in Hanover but had a large four bedroomed cabin in the woods, a reasonable distance away, where we spent a lot of the time living with nature and where we saw our first humming birds. Rosalynde and I hired a car and disappeared to explore New England for a few days and ended up on the coastline of Massachusetts and, appropriately, everywhere we went the place names were the same as England; we even found a place called Newcastle. One disappointment was when we made a long drive to Salem, the infamous town, where the inhabitants persecuted and executed innocent people charged with witchcraft in the 19th century. We ended up at the wrong Salem so that will have to wait until another visit to America.

New England is also famous for its autumnal sylvan beauty when summer ends. Believe me, there are trees everywhere you go. To be honest, I found it to be a claustrophobic part of America. There were very few open fields and the views, even at the coast, were affected by forest too. As we wouldn't be there in autumn, or fall as the Americans call it, we wouldn't see the trees changing from predominant greens to red, gold and orange as they prepared to shed their leaves for winter. We saw plenty of photographs though and it looked breathtaking.

Martha's Vineyard was something else again and eventually we all headed for the ferry, which took us across to join the Blacklows. Jim and Jane came with us, too, so there would be eight of us in one house. I began to wonder how big this island summer home was. Apparently there was a Martha and there were Vineyards but that was way back in the past when Indians lived on the island. It is now a holiday island, about one hour's journey by ferry from the mainland of Massachusetts. There are permanent islanders but not many; the summers are glorious there and the island heaves with visitors at times but we never found it over-crowded. Winters could be harsh and not many people lived

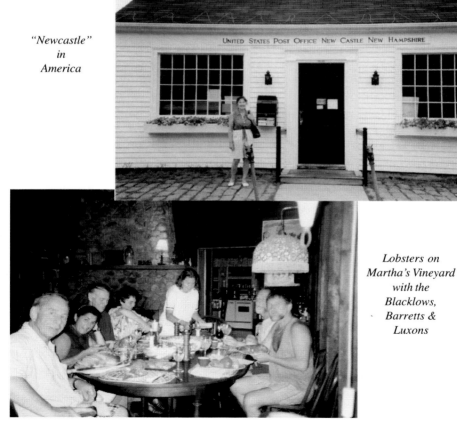

"Newcastle"
in
America

UNITED STATES POST OFFICE NEW CASTLE NEW HAMPSHIRE

Lobsters on
Martha's Vineyard
with the
Blacklows,
Barretts &
Luxons

57

there during that period. Most houses were closed down. The Vineyard's claim to fame is "Jaws", the film which broke box office records in the 70s with subsequent sequels; many of the islanders took part in them as extras.

Its other claim to fame or rather infamy was the Chappaquidich episode involving Senator Edward Kennedy and a young girl, Mary Kopekny, who drowned when Kennedy drove off the road after missing a wooden bridge, which crossed a very fast flowing stretch of sea water between two sections of the island. Kennedy survived but the incident did irreparable damage to his marriage, his career and his personal reputation. This happened in the 60s but it must still haunt him even after all that time. The original bridge has been replaced because of bizarre souvenir hunters chipping pieces off it to keep as rather ghoulish momentos.

Martha's Vineyard lived up to all our expectations. I could fill more pages with the delights of this unusual island but I will refrain from becoming carried away. We had a wonderful two weeks there adding to the pleasures of New England. The eight of us got on like a "house on fire". Ben and Sheila's concert passed successfully though we could see Ben worried about it because of his growing hearing problems. The weather couldn't have been better, hot and sunny but there was always a breeze from the sea, which kept things comfortable.

We loved the lobsters and other sea fish which we couldn't afford to buy in England and we experienced our first real clam bake on the beach one warm, balmy evening. The seafood is cooked in a huge pit dug in the sand and each layer separated by washed seaweed. The results are delicious.

The island is full of celebrities, it really is a rich person's domain. The newer houses are huge, built of wood with great verandas, most of them facing the sea, which is always dotted with white sails from the yachts. Bob and Wini lived in one of the earlier houses made of wood and clapboard like the rest. It had been owned by Bob's parents who, very wisely bought it before the island became popular. It was willed to Bob, lucky man, and they had restored and enlarged it over the years. As Bob, himself, told me there was no way he could have afforded a new property on the island at the present time. People like the Kennedys had homes there, the present President, Bill Clinton, spent summer holidays there. James Belusi, the actor, who succumbed to drugs, is buried there. His grave was such an attraction to souvenir hunters it had to be moved to a more discreet part of the cemetery.

Eventually all good things come to an end and we bade a sad farewell to our American friends. As the island slowly faded into the distance I wondered what was in store for me back in England also whether I would even visit this lovely island again.

Chapter 13
An Ambitious Project

Back in England we started work on perhaps our most ambitious venture yet – a "Proms" week. It was a crazy idea and at the same time we had just become a registered charity before leaving for America – "North East Promenaders Against Cancer" which was now official. It was divided up into a company and a trust. The company raises the money through our concerts and the profit is transferred to the Trust at the end of the year to be distributed to cancer research and patient support organisations. The amount averages an ongoing annual figure of over £50,000. A friend of mine from the Hexham Grammar School days, Peter Allan, who is a senior partner with Ward Hadaway, a big law firm in Newcastle, persuaded his partners into seeing us through the minefield of registering as a charity, a task we could not have done on our own. They very generously donated all charges which must have been considerable. All along the way we have experienced examples of support and generosity like this both from firms and individuals, it is very encouraging and heart-warming. Earlier in the year the Mayor and Mayoress of Berwick, Ian and Sheila Harris, who lived at Wooler near our cottage, rang us up to say they had been to our concerts and were so impressed with what we were trying to do they had decided the Mayor and Mayoress's charity for their year of office would be in aid of our charity. We attended a number of the events they organised during the following months and at the end of their year of office they handed us a cheque for £6,000.00 at a special ceremony at Berwick – a wonderful gesture of public spiritedness and kindness. We have been giving financial help to the North Northumberland Day Hospice during the last few years so most of the money has found its way back and is now helping people in their home area.

The "Proms" week idea was too ambitious and I really do not know why I became so carried away with it. We planned and organised a First Night of the Proms with another two concerts during the following week leading up to the annual Last Night; which was now a well established favourite in the region. This all took place at the City Hall, which meant expensive overheads and all needed sponsorship, which we found from local firms.

The amount of work involved was colossal and I regretted my impetuosity and over enthusiasm on more than one occasion. Yet the concerts were successful, each in their own way and they all made a profit. It was the "Last Night", of course, which was still the big attraction – it sold out as usual but we had attempted too much in too short a time. The best of the additional concerts was the "First Night", which was a tribute to the disappearing coalfields and coal mines of the North East. The first half was a mixture of "Geordie" and North Eastern folk music and humour and the second was a specially commissioned musical called "Fell-em-Doon", about the birth of a pit village near Ashington, Northumberland and an actual mining disaster, which took place there. It was very moving and I was in tears as were most of the audience, when, in the final moments, the cast of top local singers from the Ashington area and combined school choirs sang a haunting requiem to those killed in the disaster. They were given a standing ovation.

We received many congratulations for the Proms week but the real result, which I had hoped for did not happen. I wanted it to be an annual event and to be actually taken over by Northern Sinfonia leaving us with just the Last Night to be organised. I felt strongly that a concert series like this, perhaps spread out over a fortnight, rather than a week, could be established and there would be a demand for it provided the programmes were attractive, varied and reasonably priced. We had proved there was a demand.

It was not to be and after two more attempts on a smaller scale in 1996 and 1997 we returned to just the "Last Night" in 1998. I was saddened by this especially when we thought the First Night concert was showing all the signs of being as popular as the "Last Night". It was a complete contrast but it worked. We obviously could not repeat "Fell-em-Doon" again so we decided on a "Stars of the Future" concert bringing together all the up and coming young singers, musicians and dancers of the region together in a sparkling production of talent. And talent there was; these young people were brilliant, some of them were going on from school to colleges of drama and music while others had just graduated from them. Northern Sinfonia had just established a Young Sinfonia of budding orchestra musicians and they became our orchestra. Our soloists included a violinist from the Yehudhi Menuim School of Violinists, a harpist who was Champion of Great Britain, a young baritone graduate from the London Guildhall School of Music, graduate singers from the Glasgow Royal Academy of Music including Rachel Luxon, Ben Luxon's daughter, now following in her parents' footsteps, an Irish Dance Champion, aged 14, who stole the show with her performance based on the very popular River Dance style of dancing and many more.

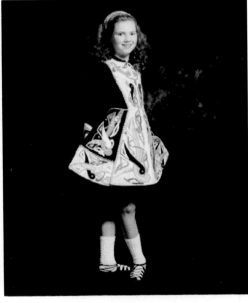

The Irish Dance Champion - by courtesy of
Gordon Swinton

The "Stars of the Future" concert with Young Sinfonia

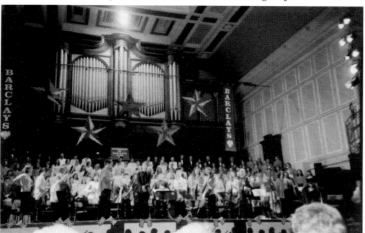

Once again and with more confidence this time, because of the Young Sinfonia's involvement, we thought Northern Sinfonia would take this over and heighten its own image in the area but it didn't come to fruition and so it became a "Last Night" only, after three interesting attempts. I'm glad we tried; they were all successful in their own way and raised a lot of money for us. We also met some more special and talented people, who were prepared to give their services to a very good cause.

Interestingly, the year after our first attempt, Sunderland Empire produced a Proms week for Sunderland including three concerts finishing with a "Last Night of the Proms". This seems to have become an established event with ironically Northern Sinfonia as the orchestra. The only difference is that it is run on a commercially run, profit making basis, not for charity. I remember being very annoyed about it and rang the Theatre Manager, pointing out that we had been going since 1990 and wasn't he jumping on our band wagon? I also pointed out that Sunderland was only about 15 or so miles from Newcastle and that was really too close for duplicating things. He replied that I did not have a monopoly on the Last Night and was in fact copying the one in London. As far as distance was concerned his concerts were to be held in summer while ours was in October, enough time between them.

I knew there wasn't anything I could do about it but I felt better for venting my feelings. Since then there are now approximately eight other "Last Night of the Proms" in the region, all of them cashing in on our idea but we were the first and they cannot take that away from us.

I have already mentioned earlier that 1995 was the 50th anniversary of the end of World War II, which was celebrated in style at our Last Night performance. It was also Suzanne Manuel's debut after meeting her in Cornwall 18 months earlier. Derrick Phoenix, an excellent tenor, also from Cornwall, had also joined the team making it, along with Ben, a Cornish "takeover". The

One Lump or Two

North East was truly linked with the South West and the "Cornish Mafia" as they became affectionately known were very quickly adopted by the audience. Suzanne and Derrick could not believe the "Geordie" welcome they received and Suzanne, whose stunning looks and personality, had the men queuing to be introduced to her during the meal at the end of the concert.

Realising how popular she was I had another of my spur of the moment ideas. Before she left for Cornwall I asked her if she would be interested in giving a small fundraising concert or recital in the following year, probably around spring if I could find a suitable venue. She was very excited about the idea and I said we'd be in touch. That was how the first Suzanne Manuel Concert came to be. It was held in May 1996 in the Newcastle Civic Centre Banqueting Hall which holds about 500 people comfortably and was a sell out.

Rosalynde and I talked about it before we made the final arrangements with her and I suggested it would be a more varied evening if it were billed as her concert but with a special guest artist in support. It would also take the pressure off performing on her own all evening.

Rosalynde agreed and Suzanne liked the idea. Our choice was a young man from Hetton-le-Hole, Stephen McElroy, the son of friends of ours. Ben Luxon had spotted his talent on a visit with us to the McElroys and had given him some coaching lessons before helping him to secure a place at the London Guildhall School of Music where Ben had first trained after Westminster College. Stephen had made great progress and we had invited him to sing at our "Stars of the Future" concert the week before Suzanne's debut. He accepted, Suzanne was happy to accept our choice even though she hadn't seen or heard him sing and we started looking for a sponsor. Later, Stephen represented Ireland in the Singer of the World Competition in 1999 which was televised all over Europe. He didn't win but he acquitted himself in great style and we were very proud of him.

As luck would have it two skiing friends of ours from the Hospital Ski Group had already expressed interest in helping us in some small way. They both ran their own company, Jim Bell owned Bell Trucks Ltd (Mercedes trucks) in Newcastle and a Mercedes car salesroom and garage in Coldstream and Jim Francis owned Francis Transport, a large haulage company in Washington. Rosalynde and I approached them with the plans and an approximate costing. They had both seen and heard Suzanne and needed no further persuasion that we had a star performer to offer and both accepted joint sponsorship of the concert and we went ahead with our plans.

It has now become an annual event with a different guest star each time and has so far raised approximately £30,000 for our charity funds. At this stage I wasn't to know that when Suzanne and Stephen performed at that concert I would have gone through a further crisis in my life and would be introducing them to the audience minus my hair for a second time after more drastic treatment – the disease had returned.

Chapter 14
A Serious Crisis – Winter 1996

By now the choice of title for this book must be clear to any reader. It came to me one day in a flash of inspiration when I actually thought I had enough material to write this sequel to "Cancer is Only a Word". "One Lump or Two" is a humorous title and very English but it has a more sinister meaning. I become confused now at trying to remember how many lumps have appeared in my body. My non-Hodgkin's lymphoma (and there are variations) has turned out to be a particular nasty one and since whatever entered my body before 1988 to trigger it all off, I am destined to be attacked by it unless a drug can be found to bring it to an end once and for all. It is not known how or why it chose me but it did and I have to just keep on fighting it if I want to keep living. Thank god, it is not hereditary so my family are safe from it that way. It also cannot be passed on to another person. It's just me in a lonely sort of way.

To date the recurrences have been low grade and responded well to all treatments I received but this next one which surfaced towards the end of January 1996 was more aggressive. Surfaced was the literal word because I began to notice a swelling near the middle of the sternum. At first I thought it a bump from a knock I might have had but it slowly became bigger and it was hard. I brought it to Graham Jackson's attention at a clinic check up and he wasn't sure about it either. Since Steve Proctor became a Professor, holding the Chair of Haematology at the University Medical School and heading the department at the RVI, Graham Jackson had become his number one Consultant. Peter Carey, who was involved in a lot of my earlier treatments, had moved to a consultant post in charge of the haematology department at a big hospital in Sunderland. I still see Peter, now a friend, because he sings in the choir at our Last Night and has always turned up to support our other functions. Graham was a worthy successor to Peter and I rate both of them as highly skilled and very caring doctors.

Graham drew Steve's attention to this phenomenon, as I regarded it, not thinking it was malignant, but when Steve booked me for a scan, misgivings began to creep in. These were confirmed when the scan showed a lymph node behind the chest wall but it had pushed or grown its way through the rib cage and that was what I had found. To be absolutely sure, it was removed surgically, at least the outside part was, and a biopsy taken. The results were confirmed and it was not low grade – it was aggressive and life threatening.

Steve said that it needed drastic treatment and I would have to go on a course of three very strong doses of chemotherapy followed by radiotherapy around the area itself. The chemotherapy would have to be spread over several weeks to allow me to recover from each of the dosages - the rescue period as it is called. I had a bone scan of the chest area in case it had spread to the rib cage but that was clear, much to my relief. During this time I would have to contend with blood counts dropping drastically, possible serious infections as my bone marrow and, therefore, immune system became hit, nausea, loss of appetite and weight and, worst of all for me anyway, I would lose my hair again. All this sounds very familiar.

I have already mentioned in my first book the very strong psychological effect hair loss means to most men. I think it is worse for men than women because they can wear a wig without embarrassment; it is part of their fashion anyway. They have, more often than not, thicker and stronger hair than men and so it is not noticeable when they wear a good quality wig. Most men's hair thins naturally as they grow older so suddenly appearing with a thick head of hair, even if it is the same colour, is very noticeable. Successful wigs consisting of thinning or fine hair styles are not possible because the membrane of the wig shows thus defeating the objective.

Fashion for men is kinder at the present time because there has been a trend to have extremely short hair styles almost to the point of being shaved in many cases. Losing it chemically though isn't quite the same because there is a noticeable difference in the pallor of the skin from the treatment and the effect of weight loss which often affects the face. Put a "skinhead" alongside a chemotherapy victim and you can usually tell the difference. Another thing I've noticed is that women can wear headscarves in all sorts of attractive and acceptable ways. Men cannot and usually revert to a baseball player's type of cap. I am no different to most men. I do not like being bald and the thought of going through all that again gave me a huge mental hurdle to overcome. If you are diagnosed with cancer, which requires strong chemotherapy, the chances are you will have to face hair loss. One consolation is that it re-grows but it takes a while. However, if the end result is that your life is saved then you have to suffer it and swallow your pride.

The only consolation prior to these events was that Rosalynde and I managed our annual ski holiday in January at Sierre Chevalier in France with the hospital crowd. The fresh air, exercise and the good company helped prepare me for what was to come.

The first treatment began on 22 February and the subsequent few days were rather unpleasant but they passed slowly but surely. What didn't help, was knowing that I would have to go through it all again at least twice. It finally reached the end in March but by then I had lost my hair and body weight. Jekyll and Hyde were back – during these periods I always felt as though I was two different people leading two very different lives.

In the middle of March I started radiotherapy at the Newcastle General Hospital. Dr Helen Lucraft once again looked after all the arrangements;

another doctor I have great respect for and I include her in my list of medical "friends". Fifteen sessions over three weeks was the prescribed treatment and I battled my way through as best as I could. That treatment on top of the chemotherapy hit me very hard but as long as I could see or feel that there was light at the end of the tunnel, I could cope with it

For exercise I did some cycling round the country lanes between Westerhope, where I lived, and Stamfordham, where there was a nice pub. One day Rosalynde was giving reflexology to a friend of ours in Ponteland and I put the bike in the car and set off from Ponteland to cycle to Stamfordham. I met some other bikers in the pub there and enjoyed the chat so much I forgot about the time resulting in a mad dash to return. I swung into the driveway at Ponteland braked, skidded, shot off the path into the rose bushes and somersaulted over them onto the lawn. Unhurt but shaken I climbed to my feet and looked around hoping no-one else had seen my embarrassing predicament. Rosalynde and her friend were looking out of the window killing themselves with laughter with no sympathy whatsoever!

Soon after that amusing episode I had lost my hair and beard and was coping with that as best I could and at the same time we had to start on Suzanne's first concert scheduled for 20th April with the young baritone, Stephen McElroy, making his debut with her. The whole evening was a great success but I had to appear without hair and beard and of course welcome the audience with a few quips and pleasantries but the reception I received from them was so heart warming I relaxed and enjoyed the evening very much.

The only thing which marred this first concert was that Alan Young, one of my close friends, had suffered a serious heart attack. He was undergoing major heart surgery so both he and Margaret were not in their usual seats that night. He eventually made a good recovery and played tennis and golf again as if nothing had happened.

I also had my SCAN just before the concert and it was clear; wonderful news once again which I was able to announce at the concert – would this be the end of it all?

Strangely enough it wasn't but in a different way because I began to notice a strange spot on the right hand side of my nose, which I just treated with cream. That seemed to work but a few days later it returned and became crustier and unsightly. I went to see my GP and he told me it was solar keratosis. This is a very early form of skin cancer caused usually by too much exposure to sun and, of course, I have spent hours outdoors walking, gardening, cycling and skiing over the years and, although 90% of the time I used sun cream, especially when skiing, I obviously hadn't taken enough precautions. It wasn't a melanoma and the cells probably hadn't turned malignant but if left untreated it could turn nasty. It then works downwards into the skin and the body and it's then when it becomes dangerous. It is particularly dangerous near the eyes and nose.

A few weeks later I was back in the RVI, this time in the Dermatology Department. The spot, which had grown bigger by then, was removed surgically by local anaesthetic so I was able to watch the process. It was painless and soon healed up. After that I made sure I was always well covered with a high factor sun lotion, I've had no problems since, just a scar on my nose. The piece removed was biopsied and had not turned malignant. Sun-seekers be warned!!

Shortly after that the Dunblane tragedy in Scotland hit the headlines and television, putting all my problems into perspective. What a dreadful, unnecessary tragedy, all those young children and staff wiped out by a madman! What a world this is at times, when, on the one side there are wonderful people helping and saving lives and on the other there are evil people destroying them and not just human beings but all that is so important to this earth of ours, the environment and the creatures which share it with us. The legacy for future generations is a very shaky one and when I think about this it always brings my thoughts around to religion.

I mentioned in my first book that when the bad news broke in 1988, I did what most people do in very frightening circumstances – I prayed to God a lot through the weeks ahead and attended the lovely little church near Kirknewton, where our cottage is situated. The combination of this and long exhilarating hours walking alone in the Cheviots were a great source of strength to me. Over the recent years though, and I'm really sorry to write this, my faith has taken quite a battering and I've thought long and hard about it.

Some people have found a very personal link with God and whether it just happened or something occurred to make it happen, I don't know. In my case I have lost that feeling, which seemed to exist during the early crisis period. Whether it is because when things look and feel better I selfishly forget about God or I have prayed for so many people over the years and seen them die that it has become too disappointing for me to bear. I have also had so many disappointments which have slowly eaten away at my faith. Whatever it is, it is a great loss because you need to have faith. When I talk to people like priests and regular church goers there never seems to be any doubts in their minds and I cannot fathom that out.

Rosalynde has this very special feeling and receives strength through it. In 1988 when she was told I only had 12 weeks to live, she refused to accept it because her inner feelings, which she believes comes from God, told her I would live – she was right and she has told me the same thing at every recurrence. Her belief in this boosts my confidence every time and jumping ahead in time to the major crisis, which was to come a few years later, she still told me the same thing. This was actually strengthened by something which took place just at the same time.

It happened in a strange way when she was returning home from visiting me at the hospital. I was in a really bad way and even her faith had been tested! She had prayed throughout it but her feelings had begun to waiver and seeds of doubt were appearing. I hadn't helped matters by telling her I wished I hadn't come out of the anaesthetic because I felt so low.

She was following a white van and this was about 9 o'clock at night and the roads were very quiet. The van just seemed to appear in front of her and when they reached a roundabout she could then see the back of the van clearly. Written in broad letters were the words "OPEN YOUR HEART". At that moment her strength and faith flooded back and she told me all about it the next day. Rosalynde, my beloved, what would I do without you?

The difference between us is that I haven't been able to open my heart. I try very hard especially when meditating and listening to Mozart, my favourite composer, but nothing happens; maybe something else has to happen before this takes place.

My own philosophy is that if there is a God and all the priests tell us there is, then why is this world in such a mess. God gave us free will so whatever happens is supposedly our own fault. After thousands of years I would have thought that, by now, God would have realised we cannot cope with free will and we desperately need help before we finally destroy this beautiful planet and everything on it.

My stomach turns every time I watch the television news and the graphic documentaries about war, atrocities, genocide, droughts and floods with epidemics of diseases, which result from it and which involve so many innocent people, especially children. How can God let this happen? Isn't it time God said "Enough is enough" and stepped in and sorted us out? I have talked to priests I know about this and even they cannot give me a satisfactory answer. Jesus Christ must have been a wonderful man and I try to model my life on his teachings – love your neighbour is the best one (that isn't always easy) and how simple it would be if we all did just that.

Power, greed, corruption and lowering of standards and morals all play big parts in this present decline and if there is any hope for the new Millennium, which is rapidly approaching, these have to be addressed by people who have the will, the strength and the power to do something about it and turn the tide before it is too late.

Enough of my religious views, back to the more worldly happenings in my life. The rest of 1996 passed without anything sinister or untoward happening. My hair was back by June and life slowly returned to normal and we felt that it was now possible to have a real break – a summer holiday in Scotland.

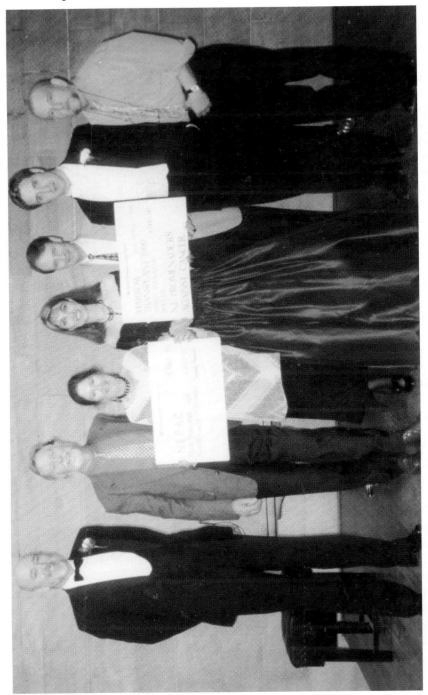

Suzanne and Anthony's first special guest star, Stephen McElroy, 2nd from right, at the Banquet Hall, Newcastle 20th April, 1996

Chapter 15
Scotland – Every Picture Tells a Story

It was only a week but it was in the beautiful Perthshire area of Scotland and we squeezed every minute of pleasure out of it. We rented a fantastic bungalow in its own little secluded valley with Alan and Margaret and John and Eileen, our staunch friends, and had a wonderful time together.

The weather was very good. I took my mountain bike and golf equipment and made good use of them. Wherever I go I always make sure I find time to look for paintings of the Victorian period and early 20th Century. Very rarely do I find anything of interest now because with the rising interest in all things Victorian, most decent objects have been snatched up by other enthusiastic collectors. Still, it's fun looking and I spend many happy hours browsing in antique shops, bric-a-brac stalls and junk shops.

Returning from a game of golf with Alan in Aberfeldy, I persuaded him to have a wander around the town with me – he knew what I was up to and I very quickly found a bric-a-brac shop. The shop was full of odds and ends, most of it rubbish. There were plenty of pictures on the wall but mainly prints and old photographs. Then, one in particular, caught my eye. I don't know why really because it was in a black chipped frame, the glass was cracked and the mounting around the picture was a dark brown piece of badly cut card – it looked completely unattractive but there was something about it which made me look twice. Alan didn't like it at all and couldn't see why I had suddenly become interested in it.

I took it off the wall and scrutinised it carefully – it was a woodland scene, rather impressionistic with a ruined house in the trees, the foreground was a clearing with a few sheep foraging for food and most importantly I could make out a sort of signature. When I find a picture like this I always try to imagine it cleaned if necessary, remounted and reframed and it is truly amazing the difference it makes afterwards. I decided to buy it if I could reduce the price. I never pay the original; part of the fun of it all is haggling with the seller.

The assistant was a rather young lady, who turned out to be standing in for her mother, the owner. The picture was priced at £38.00 and I proceeded to use all my skills and experience to knock it down pointing out the costs to me if I bought would be more than the price itself i.e. new frame, glass and mount and it probably needed cleaning. I even gave the impression I didn't really like it but was just intrigued by it.

She was a real "canny" (not the Geordie meaning) Scottish lassie and wouldn't budge on the price, which is very unusual. She finally offered a £1.00 discount but by then my stubborn streak had shot into a higher gear. Eventually we comprised. She would discuss it with her mother and see if she could reduce it to £35.00 and if I called back the following day she would let me know. At this stage I couldn't back down and had to take up the challenge, so I agreed. When we were outside the shop Alan said "I've never seen anything like that, all that bullshit and haggling for two or three pounds – it's not a decent painting either". I didn't agree.

Back at the cottage we told the others what had happened and, of course, it was not a surprise to them knowing me of old. Rosalynde and Margaret were going into the town shopping next day so they said they'd join us. This is where I use my master tactics, which has always succeeded in the past. When buying

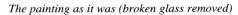

The painting as it was (broken glass removed)

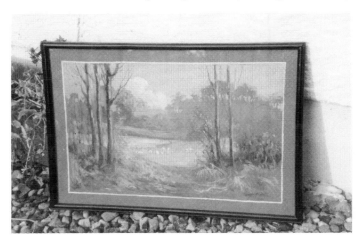

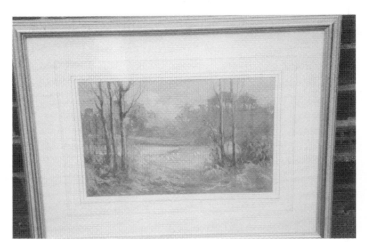

The restored painting 3 weeks later

70

a painting from an antique shop, which I've spotted I do all the initial bargaining then leave it on hold for a day with the excuse that I would like my wife to see it. Rosalynde goes in on her own and "hums and hars" in her very charming way and more often than not clinches the deal to our satisfaction – we aren't usually talking about two or three pounds though. I also wouldn't buy a picture anyway without Rosalynde seeing it first, the one exception being the oil painting of the girl, which incidentally Rosalynde loved, much to my relief.

Next day I hung around on the main street while Rosalynde and Margaret innocently browsed around the bric-a-brac shop not making anything obvious. I was impressed 10 minutes later when Rosalynde came outside with the picture and looked at it in daylight – very professional – then disappeared back into the shop. The agony of waiting to save two or three pounds – crazy but fun. Eventually they reappeared and with the picture wrapped up – the sale had gone ahead.

"How much?" I asked impatiently, as soon as we met up.

"£35.00, she knocked £3.00 off" was the reply. Honour was satisfied!

Back at the holiday cottage Rosalynde recounted the negotiations with the young lady. Rosalynde had given no indication that she was my wife or even knew me, just a passing interest in the picture and of course pointing out in her more gentle way, it needed a lot of attention.

When it was all over, the young girl said to her "I'm really glad you've bought this picture. There was an elderly (insult upon injury) man in yesterday, who spent ages pulling this picture to pieces and trying to reduce the price. He was really strange and obviously didn't like it. He is supposed to be coming back today to have another look at it and it will give me the greatest of pleasure to tell him it has been sold".

The painting returned with us to Newcastle where I spent approximately another £50.00 having it cleaned, reframed and remounted. The signature turned out to be that of a Scottish artist, W Middlemass, late 19th Century, a member of the Royal Scottish Academy, not one of the well known ones but nevertheless exhibited and recorded. The picture was transformed and valued at about £300.00 – not a bad two days' work! Even Alan liked it when he saw the finished product now hanging on our bedroom wall. I wonder what the young girl will think if by any chance she reads this. The added pleasure was squeezing a few pound out of the Scots although I would have preferred it to be a hard bitten dealer rather than a young lassie even though it was only £3.00.

It wasn't too long after returning home that we were soon in the throes of our last attempt to establish a mini Proms Series. They all sold well and the performers and programmes were excellent but it was not to be. At the end of it all, exhausted but with the usual feelings of elation, we decided to return to a "Last Night" only in the following year.

Chapter 16
Two 60th Birthday Celebrations

1997 was the year Ben Luxon and I were to celebrate our 60th birthdays, Ben in March and me in November – he always looked older than me!

We were surprised to find out that there were no special celebrations planned for Ben although it was in the newspapers and Classic FM did a birthday commemoration to him playing some of his recordings, which we taped. Ben is, however, a very private person and does not like a fuss. Rosalynde and I discussed this and decided if we could entice him up to his friends in the North, we would organise a special party for him.

This coincided nicely with Rosalynde's annual fundraising banquet at the Mandarin Restaurant in Newcastle so we decided to combine the two events and make it a surprise. Rosalynde handled the bookings and the menus, to which the response from everyone was excellent. The date was booked for 24th March, his actual birthday.

I decided to plan something special and produced a "This is Your Life" with the red book and trimmings. It was a bigger task than I thought and sometimes I curse myself for the way I always seem to jump into things with both feet, full of enthusiasm but not really looking ahead to see the consequences.

The first big task was to contact as many of his contempories in his world of opera and music as possible and ask them to send a message or preferably an audio tape. I sent letters to Dame Kiri Te Kanawa, Dame Janet Baker, Sir Simon Rattle, Felicity Palmer, Robert Tear, Seji Osawa in Japan, the world famous conductor, Sir Andrew Davies, who had conducted Ben at the Last Night of the Proms at the Albert Hall, which sparked off our "Geordie" Proms, and of course our own northern singers, Thomas Allen and Janice Cairns plus many more.

It says much for the high regard they all hold for Ben as everyone replied and most of them on tape. The next task was to produce a script using both the tapes and letters. The script had to be a pleasant mixture of fact and humour and I think it worked. I started from his early childhood days as a boy soprano chorister to his international fame as an opera singer.

Behind the scenes, we made phone calls to everyone involved with Ben and our Proms inviting them to join us. All the singers and conductors from our Last Night were able to attend except Janice Cairns who had a concert that night in London. It was kept a secret from Ben, who by this time had confirmed he would be able to come up for the fundraising banquet. Even more important for Ben was the closely guarded secret that his whole family was coming up to join us too – no easy feat for them on a working day and travelling from the south of England.

About 150 attended and The Journal did a special feature on Ben and his 60th Birthday, which was published that day and we were able to put photocopies on each table. We had a huge banner up stating "Happy 60th Birthday Ben". Everyone arrived on time except Daniel, his eldest son, who had to dash from work to Kings Cross and then catch the train to Newcastle but he was only half an hour late. Ben could not believe what was happening and was caught by surprise every time someone arrived from his illustrious past. When his family arrived he became quite emotional.

We started the evening with "This is Your Life" which, even if I say so myself, turned out well and was appreciated by everyone; the humour in it helping to put the evening into a real party swing. Ben, on our behalf, presented cheques to Steve Proctor and Tom Lennard for Bone Marrow Transplant Research and Breast Cancer; £30,000 and £8,000 respectively.

Ben & me - the "over sixties"!

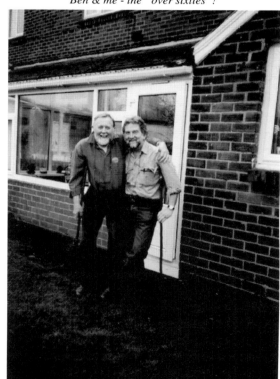

One Lump or Two

The meal was excellent and the evening ended with Ben and most of his guests becoming more than merry. Dr Peter Carey, the haematologist, who had first treated me in 1988 then set the tone with a fine and appropriate rendition of "Henry Morgan, the Pirate" and presented Ben with a bottle of rum. This was followed by Rachel, who sang "O My Beloved Father"; Suzanne sang "If I Loved You"; Daniel sang "Nessum Dorma" reaching the top notes in true Pavorotti style, even dabbing his forehead with a white hankerchief at the end; Derrick sang "A Very Special Man" and Ben staggered to his feet and sang the very appropriate "My Got Up and Go has Got Up and Went" before sinking into his seat with a beaming smile on his face.

There were other songs too but the evening finally drew to a close at about 1 am but not before Rosalynde was able to announce that, not only had it been a wonderful celebration with so many great friends, we had also raised another £1,000 for cancer research at the same time. I think we had managed to give Ben a well deserved night to remember in great company and with wonderful acknowledgements from all over the world.

My 60th birthday was not on such a lavish scale as Ben's but equally a surprise and equally enjoyable. All my close family and friends were there, with Ben making a special trip to join us.

I was completely caught out by it. I had told Rosalynde I didn't want a fuss just Marc, Roxanne, their partners and our closest friends out for a meal somewhere. It didn't quite turn out like that even though Rosalynde told me that was exactly her plan and she had a table booked at our favourite restaurant for a meal. Before that she suggested I take Marc for a drink to our Golf Club and have a chat with him about his future, which we were still worrying about. I thought it a good time to do some father and son bonding but Marc made me annoyed because he started "faffing" about as he usually does when he is going out somewhere and suddenly decided he wanted to change his trousers, then he had to iron a shirt, then he lost his tie and wallet. It was all delaying tactics, which I didn't perceive in my eagerness to have a pint of beer. We finally arrived at the Golf Club forty minutes after we were supposed to be there. The bar was deserted and that didn't help my mood, so I ordered a couple of pints and was about to knock mine back when the stewardess, Anita, came over to say hello, or so I thought. Anita is an ex-pupil of Rosalynde's and we know her very well. Her mother had recently been diagnosed with breast cancer and when she came over and asked if she could have a private word with me in the dining room, I immediately thought "Oh god, bad news – I hope not". I followed her out of the bar to the double doors of the dining room. She opened them, the room was in darkness and I followed her in. The lights flashed on and the room was full of people in party hats and holding party poppers, which they enthusiastically fired at me and began singing "Happy Birthday to You".

I had been well and truly had! Everyone close to me was there and I had a wonderful evening completing a milestone in my life, which I never thought I would reach.

Chapter 17
A Concert in Newcastle and I Find Myself Prostated

Life between those two birthday celebrations settled down to normality if that is the correct word to describe our lifestyle.

Soon after Ben's birthday party we were into organising Suzanne's second concert at the Banqueting Hall. Her guest this time was the lovely, young violinist, Sian Philipps, from Essex who had charmed everyone at our Stars of the Future concert in October of the previous year.

Suzanne, Anthony and Sian stayed at our home during the concert weekend and Sian soon became another member of our "musical family". Our house rang with the sounds of Suzanne's voice, piano and violin as they rehearsed. Rosalynde's piano is in the hallway at the foot of the staircase – not the best place for rehearsals and so our neighbours, John and Ina Wagget, offered their home for rehearsals as they too had a piano but it was in a large drawing room. Both sides of our road were entertained that weekend.

Sian was a truly dedicated, young professional and practised every spare moment. We, and I include Rosalynde, Suzanne and Anthony, were a little concerned that she was in danger of being too intense because she seemed so on edge as the concert approached and was worried and nervous about how

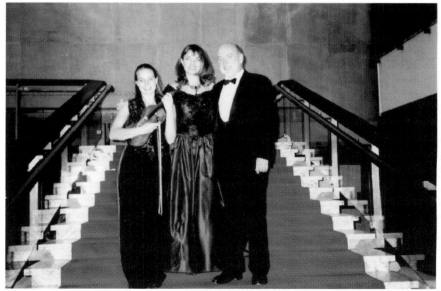

Suzanne & Anthony with special guest, Sian Philipps

she would perform. I hadn't noticed this striving for perfection when she had performed for us earlier but then I only saw her briefly at the rehearsals and after the concert at the City Hall. It is a different matter when these gifted musicians are living with you even if it is only for a short while.

I realised she was still very young and had many years of experience to come but I couldn't help feeling that the intensity and dedication she had could become too much for her if she didn't learn to relax, especially before a concert. Sian, if you ever read this, I hope you don't mind my comments – they are only meant in your best interests. I never really (and still haven't) learned to relax and I wish I had and perhaps my life may have been very much different.

In the end I think that Sian's experiences with us, and in particular with Suzanne and Anthony, helped her a great deal. They had already developed a close friendship with us and made themselves completely at home. This brushed off onto Sian and we watched her settle into the slightly crazy but humorous way of life with us and we all enjoyed each other's company.

As far as her performance was concerned, it was perfect. The three of them delighted a packed audience and what was especially nice was that at the last minute we persuaded her to invite her mother to come up and hear her play. It meant a long journey from Essex but she made it. We organised a taxi to bring her from the Central Station straight to the Civic Centre and she sat with us during the concert.

It has become a tradition now that we take our performers for a meal in a restaurant after each concert as a thank you for their generosity. That evening was no exception and we returned to La Toscana, an Italian restaurant in Newcastle near to the Civic Centre, which arranges a special table for us and dines us well.

John and Eileen Thompson, our great friends, video every concert for us and when we returned home that night we began watching it. Finally, Rosalynde and I crept off to bed exhausted , leaving our guests, who were still "high" with adrenalin, watching themselves on television.

Next morning they told us it was after 4 am before they retired to bed! I wondered how they could do that but they explained they never saw themselves perform and found it fascinating to be able to do so and hadn't wanted to stop. We had copies made for them later, which we posted on to them.

After a late breakfast our guests headed home to the South of England and we experienced the feeling of emptiness, which we always feel after a concert. We have come to know our performers so well; they are all such friendly and easy-going people that we miss them when they go.

On the medical side, I was experiencing good health and my constant body checks revealed no signs of danger. Could it be that it was gone for good? I always hoped so when things were like this but by then I had been able to make sure a tiny part of me remained conscious of the fact it could return. This was my way of avoiding being too bitterly disappointed if and when it did. It may appear as a little crack in my positiveness but I have to accept that after everything else that has happened; nothing was certain anymore.

This did not mean, however, that everything in the garden was rosy and I was, in fact, creeping slowly towards "old age". What a depressing thought! Women say they carry more crosses than men and men are one of those crosses but, physiologically speaking, they do not have a prostate. I must admit they do have "periods" and they do go through the long months of childbirth when this miracle is bestowed upon them by us men but a dodgy prostate must put all that into perspective. I first experienced it just after Suzanne's concert when we set off for a well earned break from charity work to the Cheviots, the Coldstream golf course and our cottage.

I suddenly felt the urge to urinate shortly after I had already performed that natural bodily function. Then, almost as soon as that had been completed, the same urge occurred again and I wondered what was wrong. Even the thought of it now as I am writing makes me want to go to the "loo"! This urge did not disappear as I hoped it would and persisted until my next appointment with Steve at the RVI, where I explained my predicament. After my usual check up, which was satisfactory, he concentrated on my new problem and explained about the prostate and how it sometimes enlarges as senior maturity approaches – he has a tactful way of explaining things! This enlargement puts pressure on the bladder and thus the urge to "pee". He said that some of the chemotherapy drugs, and in particular Cyclophosphamide, with which I had been treated, sometimes created problems with the prostate because of tissue scarring. There was no way of knowing without an operation, which he didn't think was necessary, at that time.

"However, we'll have it checked out" he said "I'll contact a colleague at the Urology Department at the Freeman Hospital as the RVI does not deal with this particular field of medicine. Before I left he asked me to provide a urine sample in case the problem was caused by an infection but that turned out to be negative.

True to his word, an appointment arrived a couple of weeks later for me to attend the Freeman Hospital Urology Clinic and my consultant was Professor David Neil – another Professor! Well, nothing like having the best where one's health is concerned.

Professor Neil, when I finally met him, turned out to be a charming, pleasant man and easy to talk to, which is always a good trait for a medical person. He had received a letter from Steve and had read up on my medical background. He examined me on the couch, which included another of those embarrassing rectal examinations. Professor Neil confirmed that my prostate was enlarged and I would have to go through several tests requiring further visits and he would then decide what was needed, if anything. And so I proceeded on another medical journey and, although there was always the possibility that cancer had struck again but in a different form this time, I did not have the fear and trepidation of my earlier journey.

I was curious though and more than a little apprehensive about what was to happen, both with the examination and any treatment which resulted from them. I had talked to some of my friends in the senior section of both golf clubs where I played, and I was amazed and a little comforted at how many of them had suffered or were suffering from similar prostate problems. They began to describe all the various things, which they had gone through and most of that comfort disappeared as I realised some of them were embarrassing and painful. "If only I could turn the clock back to the healthy, pain and fear free days of my youth and early middle age", I thought with a sigh at the time.

The first tests were straight forward and I began to think they had all been exaggerating just to wind me up. First I was asked not to urinate on the morning before my next appointment and when the day arrived, I presented myself with full bladder, which I proceeded to empty into a rather strange looking container. Fortunately this was done in private and my dignity was preserved. The nurse, who showed me into the room where I had to perform, explained that it was to test and measure the flow of urine and whether my bladder was completely emptied afterwards or not.

When I saw Professor Neil again he explained that the tests so far had been satisfactory for my age and he now wanted to make sure there was no malignancy and also to have a closer look at my prostate and bladder, which involved a camera. To have this done I would need to have a general anaesthetic. This required spending a day in the hospital but unless there were complications I could return home at the end of that day.

The golf seniors had not been exaggerating and when the word "camera" was mentioned I braced myself for what was to come.

Appointment day arrived, all too quickly as unpleasant things appear to do, and I reported to the clinic as arranged . After a check of temperature and blood pressure, both of which were normal, I changed into an operation gown and climbed onto one of the beds in the small ward next to the clinic and patiently awaited my fate. I was aware, at this stage, that the only way to look at the prostate by camera was via the penis and I only hoped the camera was very, very small. It is hard to imagine the size and capability of a camera, which can be inserted through a tube as narrow as the urinary tract, and then be manipulated inside the body to let the surgeon see what he has to see. Medical technology always confounds me and I never fail to marvel at how it has advanced in really what is only a short space of time since the dark days of the 19th Century.

The nurse, who was dealing with me, must have noticed my worried look and said "Don't worry, the procedure itself is straight forward and you'll sleep right through it but afterwards you will "pee" blood for a couple of days and it will feel as though you are "peeing" broken glass".

Cheerful words of comfort and I wondered where she had been trained. Do they have nurses in the Diplomatic Corps? The only comfort I had from her words was that I would sleep through it all and I kept telling myself that, as I was wheeled into the operating theatre.

It seemed only seconds had passed before I found myself back in the ward and in a daze. I remember thinking what the fuss was all about because I couldn't feel anything. However, as the anaesthetic wore off, the urge to pee increased until I told the nurse. She informed me it would be easier for me to go into the toilet rather than use a bottle and how right she was. I tottered over to the toilet with her help and I realised I was walking in real cowboy fashion as though I had been in the saddle most of my life. I had instinctively bowed my legs to ease the process of walking because of the most uncomfortable feeling in the genitalia area.

This worsened considerably when I straddled the urinal basin and tried to discharge urine. "Peeing" glass was a good way to describe it and I was shocked to see blood appear in the bowl until I remembered the nurse telling me this would happen.

"God, they must have used a Brownie Camera" I thought, "and it feels as though its still up there". There was great relief when I finished and hobbled back to my bed but the rest of my stay was most uncomfortable and lingered on for the next few days at home.

John Thompson was the first to ring me at home and after enquiring about my hospital visit he said "You haven't forgotten you are playing golf with me and Peter Jemison tomorrow have you?" I groaned inwardly because I had forgotten and I didn't really know what to say next or do about the golf. "No, of course not", I said thinking it was fortunate we were speaking by telephone and John couldn't see my expression and the bow legged way I was standing. "Right see you tomorrow. Tee off time is 2.15 pm" and that was that. Rosalynde told me I was an idiot when I explained where I was going the next day.

"They didn't remove anything" I said "except the camera, at least I think they removed it. I'm just sore really and the golf will take my mind off it".

She didn't agree but I still turned up as arranged and played some of the best golf I had played for a while. I beat Peter and halved the match with John, who, of course gave me seven shots because of the difference in our handicaps. I had a chance to beat him on the 18th green but three putted rather nervously at the critical moment to draw with him – the story of my golfing life!

They were impressed by my play, having noted my arrival and the style of walking I had adopted. They, naturally, had a good laugh at my expense when I told them what I'd been through. I attributed my improved golf to the new stance I had to adopt in keeping with the bow legs. I was also forced to slow my swing down to keep the pain between my legs to a minimum. As a good stance and a slow swing are synonymous to good golf, how could I lose? The last laugh was with me as I hobbled painfully off the last green unbeaten and unbowed.

Since then my stance has instinctively returned to the old way and my swing has speeded up. Consequently, my golf hasn't really improved although I'm quite happy not to go through the process to improve it again.

My final visit to the urology department was again with Professor Neil and we exchanged greetings. He had received the results of the endoscopy from his colleague, who had performed the operation and his report showed no malignancy present which was really good news; the bladder was fine too.

"The prostate is enlarged" said Professor Neil "and we have to decide what to do next. How are things anyway, are you still having the urge to urinate?"

As it happened, and I told him this, things had improved and although I was urinating more frequently and getting up during the night it had quietened down and I felt I could live with it. I also asked him if there were any drugs I could take to help.

"There are", he replied, "but, quite honestly, the side effects are not pleasant and I wouldn't recommend them unless there was no alternative. Why don't we leave things for a while and if you find it doesn't improve then just get in touch with me through Professor Proctor and I'll see you again?"

We left it at that and so far, although there have been times when things seemed to get worse, they have always improved after a few days. Consequently I haven't seen Professor Neil since although we have been in contact because I had a long chat with him about prostate and bladder cancer at that last appointment. Apparently men over 50 are at risk from both and although they can be cured or the cancer contained, especially if caught at the early stages, there is still a very high death rate. This led me to ask him if he was involved in researching cures and treatment for these diseases. "Very much so", was the reply and he briefly described the work he was doing at the Freeman Hospital and Newcastle University.

I then told him about our charity and asked him to send me some details of his work, which I would discuss with Rosalynde and our Trustees. He eventually sent me a breakdown of the research he and his team were carrying out and the costs involved. Resulting from this, we have been able to provide him with funds to help his work for the last three years, a total to date of over £20,000. I hope he eventually finds the big breakthrough he is looking for which will help thousands of people.

Chapter 18
A Holiday in Norfolk and an Opera in Suffolk

With all that behind me Rosalynde and I started planning a summer break, which turned out to be staying in a caravan in Norfolk with our friends from teaching days at Wideopen, John and Catherine Baugh. They had moved to St Ives where John was Deputy Head at the nearby Cambridge High School. They were keen caravaners and we had joined them on holidays on other occasions. It also coincided with Ben Luxon being asked to produce Mozart's Opera, The Magic Flute, with a cast of young, up and coming opera singers of which his daughter, Rachel, was one. This was for part of the prestigious Aldeburgh Festival at the Maltings in Suffolk. The Maltings is a huge barn-like construction with impressive outbuildings and a picturesque canal and pub nearby.

The late Benjamin Britten, the famous composer, his companion, Sir Peter Pears, and equally famous tenor, had founded the Festival converting the Maltings into a large concert hall. A fire had destroyed part of it some years ago but it had been lovingly restored. The outbuildings had also been restored and turned into the Britten & Pears School of Music in their memory. The festival was now a nationally recognised annual event.

Ben Luxon had been a principal soloist for Britten's English Opera Group in the sixties, singing there and touring with the company in Britain and abroad; Britten wrote the television opera "Owen Wingrave" for Ben, who sang the part of Owen Wingrave.

Ben was now back there but this time as a producer; the place must have had poignant memories for him. We had been there just after we were first married and stayed with Ben and his family. He had rented a house in Thorpe Ness, an unusual Victorian village further along the coast. It had been created by an eccentric but entrepreneurial millionaire towards the end of the 19th century. The idea was to use it as a holiday village

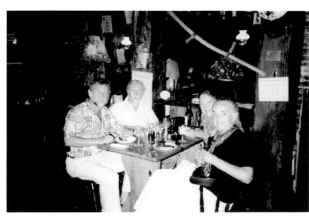

Our wedding anniversary in Norfolk with
John & Catherine Baugh

81

presumably for his rich friends and to attract middle class holiday makers. The place looked very Victorian, it was built within a stone's throw of the beach and in its centre was a boating lake with all the nautical trimmings. When we stayed there it had an air of disuse and neglect about it, a far cry from its earlier Victorian splendour. The houses, most of them of wood, needed more than a lick of paint and the whole place required a face lift. It became our home for two weeks while Ben worked at rehearsals and then the final performance, which we enjoyed very much and meeting Britten and Pears was an added bonus. In Thorpe Ness there were seven of us sharing the house and four of them children, our two and Ben and Sheila's two boys, Rachel hadn't been born then.

One day we decided to go to the beach which was only down the garden and across the road. It was quite hectic making sure we had everything, beach games, towels, drinks and food for a picnic and so on. When we finally staggered onto the beach and laid everything out Sheila said "I can't help thinking we've forgotten something". We checked everything but nothing was missing then Daniel said "Mummy where is Jonathan?" Sheila shouted in horror, "My God, we've left Jonathan behind".

Jonathan was only a few months old and had been fast asleep in his carry cot when I carried both onto the veranda. I put him in a safe place then went back inside to help the others carry things to the beach. We had all trooped past Jonathan as he lay oblivious to everything around him. Sheila ran back to the house followed by Rosalynde. Both soon returned carrying the forgotten carry cot and its contents still fast asleep as if nothing had happened.

Many years later we found ourselves back in the area to watch the youngest member of the Luxon family perform as "Queen of the Night" in her father's production of "Magic Flute". Rosalynde and I travelled from the caravan site in Norfolk, leaving the Baughs to have some peace and quiet. It wasn't too far and we were soon unpacking our things in the hotel room Ben had booked for us during our short stay.

The weather was very hot and sunny, England was experiencing a heat wave at the time. When we presented ourselves at the Concert Hall everyone, including us, was wearing the lightest and coolest summer clothes. All the doors in the place were open to circulate the air and I felt sorry for the performers, who were in full costume and wearing thick make-up.

The hall itself was packed with people, every seat had been sold but they stoically bore the heat as the cast performed like seasoned troopers rather than inexperienced but very talented young people. The audience obviously enjoyed it judging by the number of curtain calls at the end and Ben must have been very proud of them, when they drew him onto the stage to join them.

We all adjourned to the local pub afterwards for a number of long cool drinks and there we met a young singer from the cast, who was obviously enamoured with Rachel. He was a baritone and as these things seem to happen to us, he sang for us with Rachel and the rest of the Luxon family at our Millennium Concert in Newcastle in November 1999 – still a long way off! The young man's name was James Cleverton destined, like Rachel, to make names for themselves in the world of music.

We stayed on a couple of more days enjoying the sea air and sunshine including visiting Rachel, who was staying with other members of the cast in the very houses I described earlier at Thorpe Ness. We enjoyed a nostalgic tour of the place. It hadn't changed much; the boating lake was still there and the houses showed signs of improvement and were full of holiday makers.

Back at the caravan site we resumed our Norfolk holiday. This included our wedding anniversary and some very enjoyable cycling tours of the area which especially suited Rosalynde because it was so flat. On one trip we stopped at a lock-side pub along one of the broads and made a phone call from a public phone box. Two youngsters were also making a call from a second box beside us and when they had finished they handed me a wallet they had found on the shelf inside the box. They said it contained a lot of money. I opened it and sure enough there was a wad of notes which totalled over £200.00 when I counted them. I told the youngsters we'd sort it out for them and thanked them for being so honest – a rare commodity these days.

Unfortunately, there wasn't much to identify the owner in the wallet so we rang the local police and informed them of the find and told them which camp site we were staying at. We also left a note on the shelf of the phone box giving the same details just in case the owner returned.

We had drinks in the pub then cycled back to the caravan. A police car was waiting at the reception office and we stopped beside it. A policeman and a young woman came out of the office and we asked them if they were looking for us. Sure enough they were and the mystery of the lost money was solved. The woman was on holiday, touring the broads in a hired narrowboat. She had moored near the phone box to make a phone call taking all her holiday money with her for safety. It hadn't been that safe, however, as she had forgotten to pick it up afterwards. It was only after a few miles along the river that she remembered and had turned back hoping it hadn't been taken. It had of course by us but she found the note, rang the police, who very kindly picked her up and drove her to find us. She was so relieved as it was all the money she had and her holiday had only just begun. We told her about the children but unfortunately had not thought to ask their names and addresses. They may never find out that their honesty had saved a family's holiday from ruin and heartbreak.

Nothing else out of the ordinary occurred during the remainder of our holiday except for the odd bicycle puncture and we eventually returned to Newcastle suntanned and very fit.

Chapter 19
Enoch Arden, A National Tragedy, Another Proms and our First Failure

The rest of the summer passed uneventfully until Ben rang to say he was travelling to Newcastle with the Broomhill Opera Company to perform with them at the Tyne Theatre and Opera House and could he stay with us. We were delighted, of course, and looked forward to seeing him again so soon after "The Magic Flute".

Broomhill is a small but prestigious Opera Company based in London and the main performance was to be "Il Turko in Italia" by Rossini and produced by Sir Simon Callow. Ben was performing in a separate two-man show; himself and his accompanist of long standing, David Willison, a brilliant pianist. They had known and worked with each other since their student days together at the Guildhall, London. The programme was the long and very dramatic story poem by Lord Alfred Tennyson with music arranged for it by Richard Strauss – not of the famous Strauss family but a composer in his own right. Ben was to narrate this wonderful story poem accompanied by David. Both were to appear dressed in early Victorian clothes and the stage was set with period furniture.

Briefly, the story goes like this: Enoch Arden and his best friend fall in love with the same girl but it is Enoch who wins her hand. Enoch is a sailor and his friend becomes a wealthy miller. After starting a family Enoch sets off on a long voyage but fails to return. As the years go by Enoch's family is cared for by his friend, who still loves her. Eventually he manages with great difficulty, to persuade her that Enoch must be dead and she finally agrees to marry him. They do marry and have children. Enoch eventually returns after being rescued from a deserted island but he has changed physically because of his terrible ordeal. No-one recognises him and he stays at the local inn after discovering that his wife has re-married and has borne children to her new husband, his best friend.

Enoch eventually goes to the house but after seeing his wife and children through the window, she standing with a baby in her arms and looking radiantly happy, he slips away back to the inn. His health fails and as he lies dying, he tells the landlady who he is but refuses to let her bring his family to see him. He gives her a lock of hair from one of their children, who died very young. He had carried this lock ever since but wanted it returned to his wife with the message that he loved her and their children to the very end and that he understood that his friend had never meant anything but good in his actions. And so he died without them seeing him.

Rosalynde and I organised a party of our friends to attend the actual performance, which for me was one of Ben's best ever non-singing roles. I was in tears at the end and when I looked rather self consciously around, I was relieved to see most other people were reaching for their handkerchiefs too and for exactly the same reason.

If anyone ever has the chance to see a performance of Enoch Arden, I strongly recommend it provided it has the right man to play the part of Enoch. Failing that, find a book of Tennyson's poems, which contain Enoch Arden and read it. Choose the right place, a cosy room with a roaring fire and a glass of wine or something stronger to hand, oh yes, and a handkerchief too.

I said to Rosalynde afterwards that I hoped we would have the chance of seeing Ben perform Enoch Arden again at some time in the future – eventually this wish was to come true and we were to help him produce it.

Before we left the Tyne Theatre that night, its owner, Karl Watkin, came over to speak to us. Karl Watkin is a local, millionaire businessman who is interested in the art and music world. The Tyne Theatre, incidentally, used to be a seedy cinema after the last war where you could see the x-rated films of the day, if you had a trilby hat and old mackintosh! When it closed down as a cinema it was discovered that behind the film screen there was a complete Victorian stage and equipment in remarkably good condition. The old cinema was lovingly restored to its former glory as a theatre and opera house and even survived a fire several years later. It also has the great honour of being officially opened by none other than Placido Domingo himself, who was also the star of the inaugural performance.

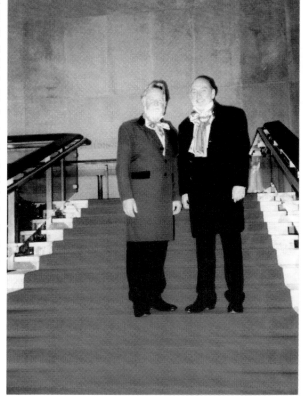

Ben & Anthony
in their "Enoch Arden" outfits

One Lump or Two

Karl Watkin was then the owner of this remarkable old building and his great ambition was to make it the home of the D'oyly Carte Opera Company, famous for its productions of Gilbert & Sullivan operas. This ambition, sadly for Karl and the area, never came to fruition.

After seeing Ben's performance and knowing about our work for cancer research, he wanted us to organise a Christmas Concert at the Tyne Theatre, which he would give free of charge. This was his reason for seeking us out that evening. He had also seen Ben perform Victorian songs with Northern Sinfonia years earlier and of course at our Last Night concerts. Ben was interested especially when Karl hoped it would be a Victorian Christmas Evening with Ben as the Master of Ceremonies. Karl became very enthusiastic at this and suggested that we meet for breakfast at a restaurant next morning which was Sunday, 31 August (I mention the date for a reason) and he would arrange for the Director of Broomhill and the Chief Executive of Northern Sinfonia to be present as he was sure they would be keen to be involved. I was amazed at the confidence and enthusiasm of the man and how he seems to feel that everyone would just fall in step with his plans. I wish I had that confidence. So we all fell in step and agreed to meet the following morning.

Everyone says that they can remember exactly what they were doing at the time that President John F Kennedy was assassinated on that fateful day in Dallas in 1963. It's true as far as I am concerned. I came home early from work, as I was due to go out again in the evening for a meeting. I switched on the television to relax and within minutes the news exploded onto the screen.

Sunday, 31 August is exactly the same and I can remember, as probably most other people can, where I was and what I was doing when first hearing about the tragic death of Princess Diana. That Sunday morning, after Enoch Arden, Ben and I left early to meet Karl Watkin and the others in Newcastle. Rosalynde had decided there was too much to do at home to be able to join us. As soon as we entered the restaurant, which was warm and smelling deliciously of coffee, bacon and toast, Karl Watkin rose to greet us and then said "Have you heard the news?" We hadn't because of the rush and my car radio wasn't working. Then he dropped the bombshell and told us about the dreadful accident in Paris, which had resulted in the death of one of Britain's best loved and controversial figures. Princess Diana, at the time of her life when she seemed to be finding the happiness which had hitherto eluded her, was dead. The media would probably turn it into a circus and she would become as much a celebrity in death as she was in her life.

The meeting during breakfast was over-shadowed by Karl's news but we talked things through between bites. Mark Dornford-May of Broomhill Opera and John Summers of Northern Sinfonia were both present and responded positively to Karl's enthusiasm. We now had high hopes of a successful fundraising event especially with the Opera Company and Northern Sinfonia becoming involved. Each of us took responsibility for part of the organisation. Ben was to plan the programme, Mark would provide singers and costumes, John the musicians and I was to handle sponsorship and publicity. It seemed, as if it couldn't possibly fail., but it did. People did not "deliver the goods", things that were promised to happen did not happen even though protests were made and meetings were arranged.

In the end and by the time it was only a few weeks from the proposed date, just before Christmas, I took it upon myself, having talked to Rosalynde, Ben and the Trustees of our charity, to cancel it. It was disappointing but after the decision was made both Rosalynde and I felt relieved. Our First and Last Night concerts in the October had been successes, each in their own way but it had been the usual hard but rewarding work and a third concert so soon after was realistically too much for us to carry.

At the same time we were also experiencing another failure – we had failed to convince the people, who were in the right places, to take over the "Proms" concert series, which we had hoped to achieve. The Stars of the Future II, as we called it, was every bit as good as its predecessor in 1996. Rachel Luxon, Ben's daughter, accompanied by a young American baritone called Nathanial Webster, known to us, and his friends as "Nate", stole the show this time. They were both in the middle of their courses at the Glasgow Royal Academy of Music and were so good we asked them straight after the concert if they would be Suzanne's special guests at her next concert for us in 1998, which they immediately accepted. This meant that we would only have two concerts to organise and worry about next year as we had already reached the decision to go back to just the Last Night concert in October.

A wise decision bearing in mind that the proposed Christmas concert had turned into a nightmare and cancelling it had been the right decision in the end.

Fortunately we didn't have the same problem with the big October concert, just the opposite. We had a full house again and all our stars appeared and with them we introduced our first instrumental soloist, Bradley Creswick. Bradley is a well known and greatly admired violinist. His main role is as leader of Northern Sinfonia but he is a solo concert performer in his own right and does regular master classes on Classic FM and elsewhere. He added a new dimension to the programme and has become a regular ever since. The lighter side of the programme this time was the Toy Symphony with the audience bringing various toy instruments with them and joining in under the humorous direction of the soloists who even had an appropriate instrument. This was followed by a tribute to Noel Coward and Ben Luxon's rendition of "Nina from Argentina", dancing as well as singing had the audience in stitches.

Chapter 20
1998 – Rosalynde Reaches a Milestone but has an Accident

I found it hard to believe, on looking back at 1997, that the lymphoma had not returned and the tiny glimmer of hope reappeared – maybe this time it would not occur again but I've said this before and I knew deep down not to become too carried away.

The first day of 1998 found us at our cottage. We had a quiet celebration on New Year's Eve just ourselves and our neighbour, Emily, but in front of a warm fire and with a bottle of Champagne. Next morning, the weather was just like a good summer's day so we rose early and after breakfast headed for the golf course at Coldstream. We were the only people there, everyone else was sleeping off the effects of Hogmanay. We took advantage of it, playing each hole leisurely and absorbing the sunshine and peace of the place.

When we returned to the clubhouse people were arriving for Sunday lunchtime drinks, some of them looking the worse for wear. In comparison we were positively glowing with the fresh air and exercise and decided to do the same the following year.

Later that month another celebration took place – this time it was Rosalynde's 60th Birthday. She told me emphatically that she did not want any surprises, just a gathering of Avril, her sister, and family, Joan and Lara and all our friends and that is exactly what happened. I did work hard to make it special, something she really deserved.

All our friends are from the 60s and 70s era so I spent a long time going through all our records and CDs extracting short but identifiable pieces and put them all onto one tape. This was to be used for a quiz during the party. When everyone arrived each person had a name or title pinned to their back. The names were partners and without looking at backs they had to ask questions around the room to find their matching partner – it was a good ice-breaker and set the party off to a cheerful start.

After a delicious meal, not all prepared by me, Roxanne, Marc and friends helped too – we presented Rosalynde with her presents and sang "Happy Birthday" as she cut her cake.

I gave her a new set of golf clubs to which was added a golf bag from John, Eileen, Alan and Margaret. Most of the other presents were also connected with golf – it was just as well she enjoyed playing.

Finally, I dressed her up in what I described as an over sixties survival kit, which consisted of a grotesque wig, false teeth (plastic), horn-rimmed specs, a whistle and compass, a tube and colostomy bag (not the real thing but realistic enough) and a notice to hang around her neck which said "Please help me I'm over 60". It was hilarious even though she was embarrassed, but I think she enjoyed it. Her audience certainly did.

Roxanne's birthday a few weeks later was a much more subdued affair but just as enjoyable. She was experiencing a hectic but ultimately rewarding time in her life with her partner, Russell, house hunting. They finally found a house in our village of Westerhope, a place she said she would never return to but they loved what they found and we agreed with them. It was a stone built house, one of five in a terrace, which had originally been farm cottages towards the end of the 19th Century. It had been modernised, had a small but pleasant garden and importantly, a garage. Their offer was accepted and they prepared to move into their first real home.

Marc, on the other hand, was experiencing a dreadful time in Edinburgh. The firm he had helped to establish after graduating with a Master's Degree had been taken over and the firm responsible had then gone into liquidation – the erratic business world at its worst! He hadn't been paid for the past couple of months so we had to send him money to help him out. His type of work was multi-media technology and Edinburgh was not progressing in that direction so there were very few jobs available which suited his qualifications. London was the place for the experience and, after a bad work experience in Edinburgh it was there he finally went, securing a Consultant's post with the Stationery Office, which handles all the government's publications. His partner, Catherine, had to stay in Edinburgh because of her work as a translator so it meant a great deal of travel and expense which eroded much of his exceptionally good salary but if he wanted this good working experience it was something he had to do.

Healthwise, I was reasonably well except for an unexplained loss of appetite but my February check up at the RVI showed nothing amiss. Rosalynde was not her usual healthy self, however, and was experiencing pains down the left side of her head and when she swallowed she felt as though there was something stuck in the throat – a lump! Both were very worrying especially the lump but after checks with our G.P. and then a consultant, they couldn't find anything out of the ordinary and both were put down to stress, of which she had more than her fair share. These symptoms still bother her and can be very painful and uncomfortable at times. If it is stress then I must bear responsibility for that and it is a hard cross to carry. Perhaps when this is all over one or both symptoms will disappear – I hope so.

Fundraising for cancer research, always with us, was starting to move up a gear. Rosalynde had her annual Chinese banquet at the Mandarin Restaurant in Newcastle, which went very well, raising over £1,000 and we began planning our third concert with Suzanne Manuell at the Civic Centre Banqueting Hall. We had one break from charity work when we headed to France on the

One Lump or Two

Newcastle General Hospital Ski Club's annual ski trip. This time it was to Val D'Isere, a top resort linked to Tignes, another resort, and both had excellent facilities and a good snow record over the years.

We had a great time until the second last day when the weather was hot and sunny, perhaps too hot. After skiing the runs in Val D'Isere, where we were based, we crossed over the mountain and dropped into Tignes and then up to its highest point. From there it was a black run (the steepest) changing into a red and eventually a blue as we approached the village. We had no difficulty with the black and red runs and Eileen and I raced off ahead once we hit the blue which was a relatively easy but still exciting run. Her husband, John, stayed with Rosalynde. John and Eileen Ellwood are both nursing officers at the RVI, Eileen is a Casualty Sister and John works in the operating theatre – plastic surgery is his speciality. Both are very good skiers and we have enjoyed their company on many skiing holidays.

After dropping about a mile down the blue run, which became rather heavy going because of the warm temperature, the piste swung into a steep corner. Rounding it I could see a number of pistes in the far distance so decided to stop and wait for Rosalynde and John. We waited and waited but they didn't appear and eventually I stopped a passing skier, who was shouting in English to her friend. I asked her if she had noticed an accident on the run down. She had, one skier down and another helping. A pair of skis were crossed and stuck into the snow above them, the international sign of an accident or hazard to skiers.

I described the clothes they were wearing, Rosalynde's was easily identifiable and she thought it fitted the person on the ground. I thanked her and asked Eileen to stay where she was while I skied down then caught the lift back up to where they were.

When I finally reached the spot there was no sign anywhere of Rosalynde and John so I skied back down to Eileen. John was with her but no Rosalynde. He explained that she had fallen, blaming the sudden change from snow conditions higher up the mountain to the softer but heavier snow melting in the sunshine. This often happens – slopes higher up the mountain might be steeper but the air temperature and therefore the snow remains constant. Lower down, where it can be much warmer, especially on a sunny day, it is very different and even experienced skiers can find it difficult. This is what happened to Rosalynde and unfortunately one of her ski bindings did not release causing her leg to twist as she fell.

John had called for help to a passing ski instructor who had radioed for assistance. Rosalynde had her first experience of being taken down the mountain in a "blood wagon" as it is called. This is a specially designed sledge where the "victim" is wrapped up like a cocoon for the rather bumpy and ignominious journey behind an experienced mountain skier. He is ahead of the sledge between two arms attached to it – rather like a horse and cart, without a horse or wheels.

John knew where she was being taken and we followed him down to the village and located her in the casualty department of the local hospital. She was actually being treated when we arrived so we sat outside in the sunshine until the nurse called us in. I was very relieved to see her smiling but she had torn her knee ligaments rather badly and had the x-rays to take back with her to England. The doctor had told her nothing was broken, rest and then exercise was the answer but to report to the hospital on her return to England. The ambulance was waiting to take her and us back to the hotel, a journey of about 10 miles around the mountain to Val D'Isere.

Rosalynde, by this time, had told us that the charges so far were £327 to be lifted on the mountain, which she couldn't pay. They were also holding her skis at the ski school until she paid for the sledge etc. Fortunately, John had his Barclaycard. What an advert that would make! He settled the bills for us foolishly thinking we would pay him back in England –only joking!

That was the end of skiing for Rosalynde but at least it was the second last day. Conditions changed dramatically anyway on the last day. Strong, bitterly cold winds blew most of the snow off the pistes leaving them very icy and extremely difficulty to ski. Most people who ventured out didn't ski for very long. I lasted about three hours with David Belcher, who organised these weeks with his wife, Cathy.

Rosalynde had an uncomfortable journey back to England and is still undergoing physiotherapy on her knee and we haven't skied since. We miss it and the crowd of friends we made very much. I've taught many of them to ski over the years. One member of the group told me he could always recognise people from the group on the pistes as they skied just like me – I hope that was a compliment.

Rosalynde's 60th Birthday Celebration

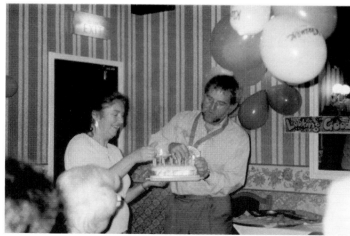

Chapter 21
Suzanne's Concert and a Double Shock

Not all our holidays in Cornwall were spent on fun and relaxation, we did actually do some charity work even that far from home. It was an excellent opportunity to discuss the programme for the May concert with Suzanne and Anthony but it was much more enjoyable than over the phone or by letter. They were also able to play and sing some of the suggested songs we didn't recognise by name, which was an added bonus. Suzanne's two guests this time, Rachel Luxon and a young American, Nate (Nathaniel) Webster, both in their final year at the Glasgow Royal Academy and both had sung so well for us at the last "Stars of the Future" concert in the previous October, which was why we had invited them to return to Newcastle.

The break was just what we needed and after a few days of readjusting to the daily chores of home life we started working on the concert which was scheduled for 10th May, only a few weeks away.

During all this time I still worried about the lump under my arm which no-one except Rosalynde and Steve Proctor knew about. It showed no signs of disappearing and I thought it was growing. I mentioned this to Steve on my next visit to his clinic and he decided the only way to find out was to have a biopsy, which he would arrange.

Once again I found myself under the knife of the very skilled surgeon, Tom Lennard, this time as a day patient. Rosalynde took me in by car and left me in his capable hands and returned for me when I recovered from the anaesthetic some hours later. The first thing I remembered after coming round was the soreness under my arm where they had removed all or some of the lump to be sent to the pathologist for confirmation one way or the other. Actually I knew before that result because Tom's registrar came to talk to me beforehand and told me they were certain it was lymphoma.

I didn't tell Rosalynde until we returned home and her first words were "Don't worry love, we've been there before, we won on those occasions and we'll win again, trust me".

I did, but I knew there was another long, uphill stormy road to face before I arrived at the end of it.

We talked for a long time that evening, sitting on the settee, holding hands and both trying to give each other the strength to face another uncertain future. Against her will, I made Rosalynde promise not to tell anyone especially Marc and Roxanne. She was very much against it but I said it would help me to cope better not having to worry about them and the rest of my friends. Rosalynde also knew I hated being treated as a sick person and sympathy, no matter how well intended, did nothing to help me remain firm in my resolve to regain normality in my life.

And so very few people were to know that throughout the build up to Suzanne's concert I went through 15 sessions of radiotherapy on the area under my arm and then half way through another lump appeared on my neck at the front below my chin. I had just returned from a visit to the RVI supposedly to see Steve Proctor, only to find out he was ill and not at work. I saw his second-in-command, Graham Jackson, with whom I'm completely comfortable. It was a discussion really, not a check-up in the usual way; simply to find out how I was coping with the radiotherapy, which was being carried out at the General Hospital, not the RVI. So the second lump was not noticed until I returned home. Rosalynde was upstairs when I entered and I shouted, "I'm home", and she came down to greet me. Unbelievably, as she came downstairs I felt an uncomfortable feeling in my neck and by reflex my hand just strayed up there as I returned her greeting. A greeting which I didn't finish. I leaned weakly against the wall in shock and almost knocked a picture from its hook.

"What's wrong?" Rosalynde's words came through the shock waves, bringing me back to reality. Shock turned into anger as I felt deeply the unfairness of it all and I just straightened up put my arms around Rosalynde and just held on to her. She knew immediately something was dreadfully wrong and she spoke soothingly into my ear as she returned my hug.

"What's wrong darling? Tell me please". It was just like pressing a button to repeat something over and over again. How many time has she heard this now?

"Oh god, you'll never believe this but I've just found another lump, on my neck this time. Here, feel it" and she did, confirming that it wasn't just my imagination.

"Why haven't I spotted this before now or

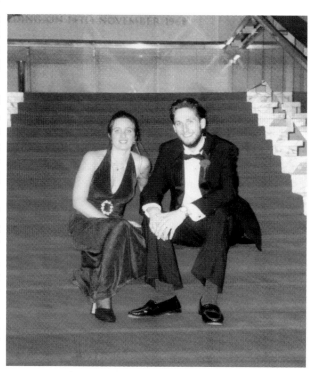

Suzanne & Anthony's special guests,
Rachel Luxon & Nathaniel Webster

93

anyone else for that matter with all this treatment under my arm going on?" I asked this more to myself than to Rosalynde. "I've just come back from the bloody hospital!"

"How quickly can these damn lumps appear; it is not instantaneous surely?" was my next question, which, of course, neither of us could answer.

As the shock wore off and reality took over, I telephoned the RVI and spoke to Graham, who fortunately, was still at the clinic and he told me to come in straight away. I did just that and he confirmed my fears as soon as he had looked at it and felt my neck.

"George", he said, "I know how you must be feeling but I'm sure it is another low grade tumour like the one under your arm. I'll inform Dr Lucraft, who is overseeing your radiotherapy treatment at the General and she will re-adjust your treatment to take care of this little fellow".

His calm, gentle approach to my situation eased the turbulence going through my mind and I left for home feeling reassured and more relaxed than on my journey in. Sure enough, at my next visit to the General Hospital Dr Lucraft spent some time with me talking about this new set back.

"I've had a long talk with Dr Jackson", she explained, "and he had been in touch with Professor Proctor, who as you know is ill at home at the moment. We have decided to treat the whole lymphatic area from both sides of the your neck to the area under both arms. This will eradicate any thing else which might be lurking there".

"It means extending your treatment by a few more weeks but it is the best possible answer for this particular situation".

Who was I to argue with the experts?

I forgot to mention earlier that exact measurements are made on the surface of the body to be treated by radiotherapy. This is to make sure the rays do not go beyond the area to be treated thus damaging healthy cells. You are asked not to wash the area to be treated in order not to remove the markings; washing also makes the skin more tender than it needs to be. However, wearing clothes and perspiration tends to wipe off some of the marks so they often have to be renewed by the radiographer.

It was easy to hide these marks when they were just under the armpit but not so when purple lines and crosses appeared on my neck. When this more drastic treatment began I had great difficulty in hiding the marks on my neck from inquisitive eyes. None more so than my daughter, Roxanne, who was always quietly scrutinising me whenever she suspected that my health was not as it should be. It was easier with Marc because he was living a long way from home at the time. Eventually Roxanne spotted the marks and honed in like a spider on a fly. I've tried hard to remember what it was that I made up, something about experimenting with a blue carbon pencil to mark a line on my neck to change the shape of my beard, I think. Whatever, it only half fooled her and

I'm sure she knew but respected my feelings and quietly went along with it.

Rosalynde told me a long time afterwards that she was actually furious with me and my obstinacy in trying to keep it all bottled up but I stuck to my guns, which were exactly the reasons I gave earlier in this chapter.

I discovered the second lump several days before Suzanne's concert which took place on 9th May. Life had been very hectic in the build up to the concert and dashing to the hospital for treatment made me feel very tired.

The concert itself took my mind of it and it was enjoyed by everyone who was there. Suzanne and Rachel looked radiantly beautiful and sang very well. I could tell Rachel was nervous at the beginning, not surprisingly, but she soon settled down and won the hearts of the audience. Her mother, Sheila, was there having travelled up from Canterbury but Ben was working in London and just couldn't make it, although he did send a message which was read out in my opening address. Nate, the young American baritone, resplendent in black evening suit had a wonderful voice. He was tall, bearded and had a very good stage presence. There is no doubt that both he and Rachel will go far when they finish their studies in Glasgow.

Next day everyone departed on their different ways and we were left in relative peace though we were sorry they all had to leave so soon. There was always a feeling of anti-climax the day after a successful concert.

This did not last long, however, because my treatment started again on the Monday so life returned to normal, if that's the way our lives could be described! As the radiotherapy treatment came to its close Steve Proctor returned to work and I saw him again after the last dose of radiotherapy. Two things happened about that time. Firstly, Steve rang me about a new drug, which was particularly suitable for non-Hodgkin's patients. This was the phone call I mentioned at the very beginning of this book and was the main stimulant for writing it. The drug was called Rituximab which is a monoclonal antibody against CD20, an antigen expressed by the lymphoma cells in a tumour. Preliminary studies had shown successful response from some patients with low grade non-Hodgkin's disease.

Steve told me that Roche, the drug company which produced it had offered him a limited supply of the drug to test on his patients. He had selected three and I was to be one of them, if agreeable. The other good thing about this drug was that it had very few side effects and patients did not lose their hair. Steve wanted to try it out on me as a back up procedure when I finished the radiotherapy treatment, which, was only a few days away. Of course, I jumped at the chance and arranged to meet Steve that same week to discuss arrangements. At the time I thought this was a wonder drug and something which could bring all my health problems to an end.

The other thing which occurred was from another phone call about the same time. It was from Alan Fairnington, a television producer with the BBC based at Newcastle. He told me the BBC was interested in his suggestion that a follow up programme be produced about how I was healthwise, how I was coping with things and, of course, the continued annual success of our North East Last Night of the Proms. The BBC had already produced a programme which was called "George & the Geordie Proms". It was half an hour long and shown on BBC2 North in 1992, a month after our 3rd Proms, which took us to £100,000, a target we had set earlier. The programme had covered just about everything Rosalynde and I had gone through together including excerpts from the concert rehearsal and the concert itself. Alan's idea was to produce a sequel to this in much the same pattern as the first and again ending with shots from the concert. We agreed to this and the filming was spread over the summer keeping the final shots until the concert in October.

We weren't exactly veterans at this but the earlier experiences helped us and we were less nervous during the shots that were taken. These included Rosalynde and I playing golf at the Hirsel Golf Club near our cottage where we had the course to ourselves as the course was closed due to flooding. The spring and early summer of 1998 was very cold, wet and miserable. The Club Captain gave us special permission for the filming, even joining us for the two holes we played.

Alan also brought the camera crew into the RVI and filmed one of the four sessions I had when the drug Rituximab was being intravenously fed into my bloodstream. Each of these sessions lasted between six and seven hours and I was monitored throughout by Phil Mounter, one of Steve's team, and Carol Richardson, who had helped to nurse me through my bone marrow transplant in 1989. She was now in charge of the after care of patients when they have had transplants – a very responsible position.

Rosalynde was with me all the time too and we got to know them both well as a result. We even had them checking and posting tickets during the last session for the Proms. My bed was covered with tickets and envelopes. Not exactly normal practice for them but it certainly helped to pass the time away.

All this took place during the summer and it ended with a scan, which showed I was completely clear. It was a marvellous feeling for me and for everyone else close to me and I thought at last it might be over for good – no more worry and no more fear.

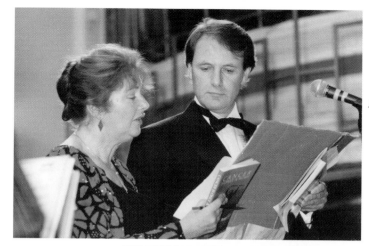

Rosalynde & Steve Proctor introducing Book One to the audience

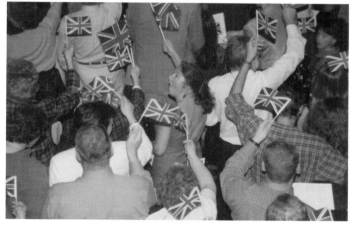

Rosalynde waving the flag - Rule Britannia

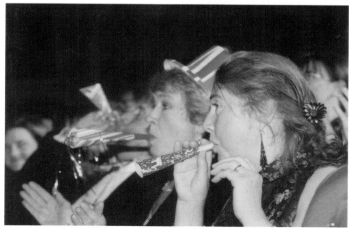

Rosalynde & Hilary Phoenix (Derrick's wife) accompanying the arrival of the Queen of Sheba with the rest of the audience

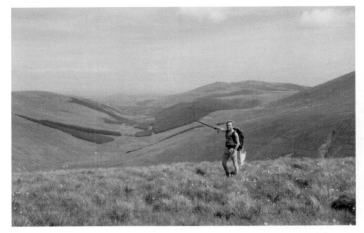

Beside the Border fence between Scotland and England pointing to Kypie Hill where the cottage is situated

Ben Luxon, Tom Allen, Janice Cairns & Suzanne Manuell in full voice at our last Proms of the Millennium (October 1999)

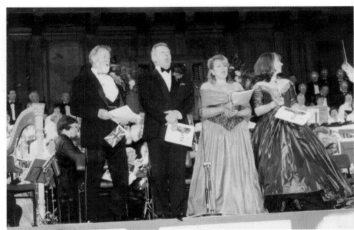

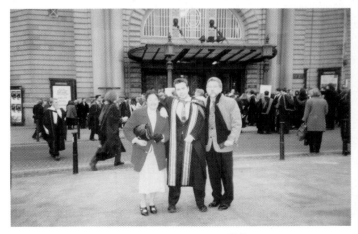

Marc's M.Sc. Graduation in Edinburgh with proud parents

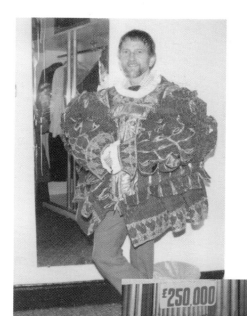

George wearing Ben Luxon's costume at the London Coliseum production of Falstaff starring Ben Luxon & Janice Cairns

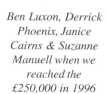

Ben Luxon, Derrick Phoenix, Janice Cairns & Suzanne Manuell when we reached the £250,000 in 1996

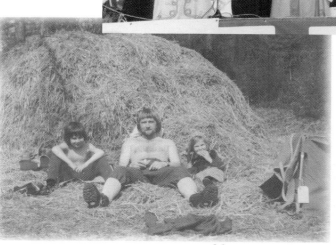

Picnic time with Marc & Roxanne in the Austrian Tyrol (1974)

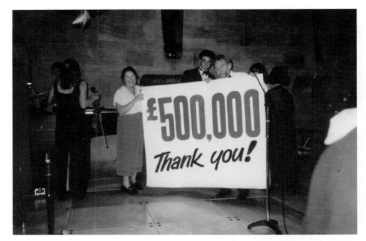

Finally reaching the £500,000 target at the Millennium Concert, November 1999, at the Banquet Hall, Newcastle Civic Centre

A Proms finale with the packed audience enjoying the balloons

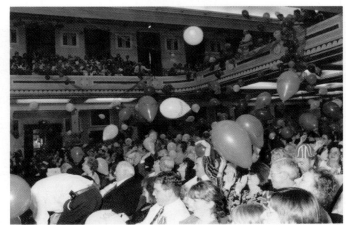

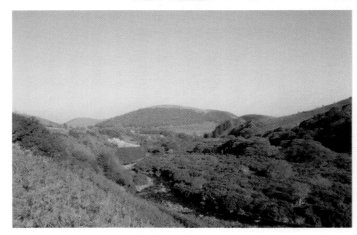

College Valley, (Cheviots) in Autumn

*The Walker family
at the Geordie
Proms*

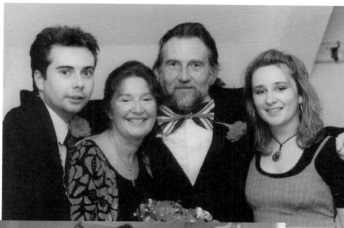

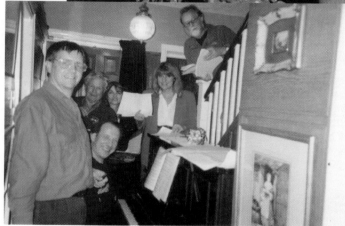

*Rehearsing in our hallway for the proms concert - a tight squeeze for Len, Richard, Derrick,
Suzanne, Janice & Ben*

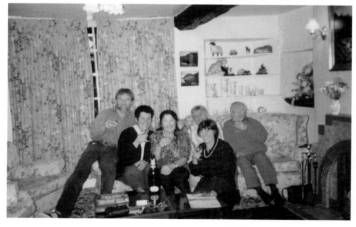

*Recovering after the
Proms at High
Lodore Farm,
Cumbria*

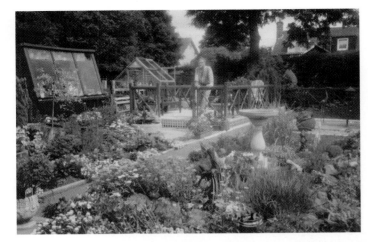

Our garden finished in time for our 40th Wedding Anniversary - 12th August 2001

Ben's 60th Birthday - Rosalynde presenting cheque from NEPAC to surgeon, Tom Lennard, for his Breast Cancer Research Appeal, R.V.I.

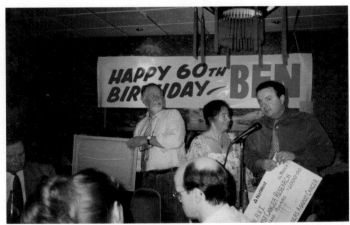

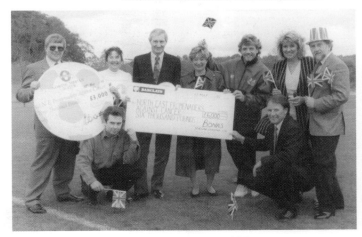

Janice Cairns & Kevin Keegan presenting cheques to NEPAC at Newcastle United's Training Ground

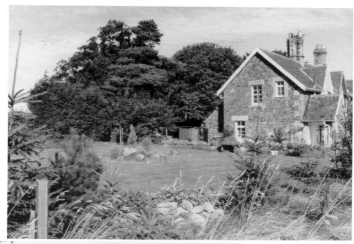

Our cottage and garden near the Scottish Borders

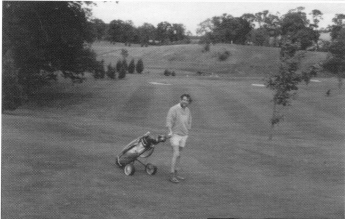

My hole in one at the Hirsel Golf Course, Coldstream; the tee box is on the top of the slope in the background with the green below

Sister Lorna Rennick, the "Angel" of Ward 8

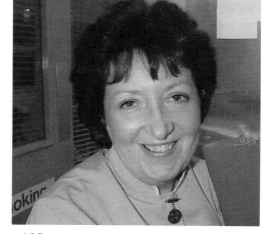

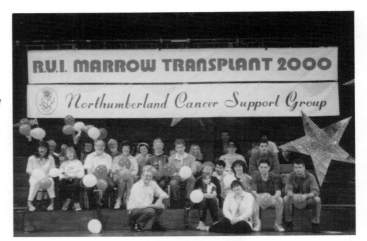

Our wonderful band of helpers who turn up at every concert

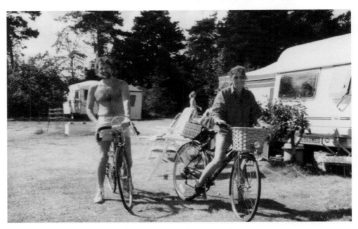

Cycling on our Norfolk holiday

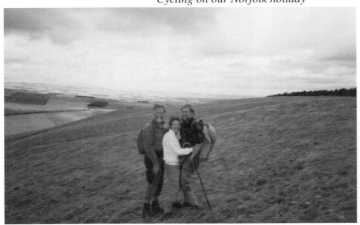

Filming "George & the Geordie Proms" on the edge of the Cheviots with Ben Luxon and Rosalynde - BBC TV, Close Up North

Chapter 22
Tragedy in Cornwall

Basking in this euphoric feeling plus the fact that the weather had picked up and we were experiencing a mini heat wave made us decide to re-visit our special musical friends in Cornwall. After a few phone calls to Ben, Suzanne, Derrick and Anthony, we packed the car and headed south. We had promised Anthony and Sarah we would stay with them on our next visit to Cornwall and so we headed there but we had promised to spend some time with the others too.

Anthony and Sarah have a lovely house overlooking the River Truro's estuary and what was even more attractive, we discovered they had a snug, little pub next door which sold good beer and food. Golf was on the cards too and we were looking forward to seeing Ben's new extensions to his house and garden. All the ingredients were there for a terrific holiday.

But it was not to be. Tragedy struck on the fifth day of our visit. Before that I enjoyed some golf with Anthony on his local course while Rosalynde went shopping in Truro. Next day we played tennis with Sarah in Truro where we were joined by Derrick Phoenix and his wife, Hilary, and their lively gold retriever, Jamie. After tennis we all retired to the Swan Inn on a bend of the Truro river and had lunch together outside on the veranda in warm sunshine. During the meal everyone was in agreement to have a barbeque party the following evening at Anthony and Sarah's house. On our return to the house Anthony rang Ben and Suzanne, who were able to join us, Ben with his mother and Suzanne with William and their two children. A gathering of the Cornish "Mafia" with their two "Geordie" friends and no audience this time, just some good food, wine and music. Anthony also arranged a morning's round of golf, a foursome, Cornwall against the North East, which I am delighted to report was won by Rosalynde and myself. The critical moment in that game was when Anthony very chivalrously gave Rosalynde a six foot put. He was so intent on beating my score on that hole that he forgot Rosalynde had a shot there. We all ended up with a five but with Rosalynde's shot it made her four and she won the hole for us. Anthony's golf was never the same after that and we won the match by a single hole. Well done the "Geordies!"

In the afternoon we started preparing the food and the barbeque. It was still a glorious day and it looked as though it was going to be one of those warm, balmy evenings when you can sit outside until very late – a rare occasion in our part of the country.

When everything was ready we all gathered outside for gin and tonics on the patio overlooking the estuary. We just sat there absorbing the peace and beauty of the scene in front of us. The tide was in, a yacht sailed passed us up river to its moorings, various sea birds were flying around making contented calls to their mates and the sun's rays were just catching the water producing shimmering light. Only two people and a dog were missing, Derrick, Hilary and Jamie. We just thought something had held them up so no-one was really concerned. We sat and chatted for a while and just as we decided it was time to light the barbeque we heard the telephone ring inside the house. Anthony, being a GP as well as an excellent musician dashed in to answer it. We carried on with the preparation until Anthony reappeared and I could tell by the way he looked that something was wrong but I wasn't prepared for the bombshell he dropped on us.

"The call was from one of my colleagues at the practice", he said in a quiet but clear voice, "Derrick has just been rushed to hospital by the air ambulance but he was found to be dead on arrival".

We stood there facing him, stunned for a moment then someone, I don't know who it was, asked the question everyone must have been thinking, "What happened, was it an accident?"

"Apparently Derrick took Jamie for a walk on their favourite beach. Derrick had gone in for a swim. After he came out and was drying himself another chap walked by with his dog and they started talking. He then left Derrick but something made him turn around and he saw Derrick collapse onto the sand. He rushed back, saw there was something seriously wrong and ran to the nearest telephone and called the emergency services. The helicopter arrived very quickly and rushed Derrick to Truro Hospital. From what I gather Derrick must have died instantly – there was nothing they could do for him. It was probably a massive heart attack but we won't know the true facts until they perform an autopsy".

For a moment there was silence then Anthony continued "I thought I'd tell you all just before I speak to Hilary, who has been taken home from the hospital. She dashed there as soon as they informed her. I think she collected Jamie at the same time".

Sarah went into the house with Anthony to telephone Hilary. Rosalynde ran in after them and suggested they ask Hilary to drive over to join us. She thought, quite wisely, it was best to be with family or friends at a time like this and their family were all living away.

After a few minutes they returned and said Hilary would join us as soon as she had made some phone calls to her immediate family. She very bravely joined us about an hour later. By this time we had decided not to overwhelm her with questions and sympathy but to let things happen naturally and with ease, if that was at all possible. We were very apprehensive but it was Hilary, herself, who made it easy for us. She arrived with Jamie who jumped up to greet everyone, wagging his tail in pleasure; oblivious to the situation but helping to break the ice in his usual exuberant way. As each of us escaped from his attentions, we gave

Hilary a warm hug of friendship and sympathy, each murmuring words, which were well intended but extremely inadequate under the circumstances. What can anyone really say to make up for the loss of a loved one and, especially, in the way it happened, so sudden and unexpected. Hilary would have watched them leave their home for their walk, not to see her husband alive again. I can't think of anything harder to bear than that.

The evening, I'm glad to say went ahead almost as though Derrick was still with us. Of course, there wasn't the usual noise of laughter and jollity you'd expect to find at a barbeque. He was certainly the centre of conversation; warm, friendly and quiet conversations. Everyone had something to tell about the memories he had left behind and I like to think that it helped to ease some of Hilary's pain and anguish.

When it was time to leave, Rosalynde and I offered to stay overnight with Hilary until her sister arrived from London the next day. Hilary accepted our offer and we packed our night things and followed behind in our own car. It was late when we reached her home and although we were tired it was obvious that Hilary was still in shock or back in shock after the brief break in the company of friends at the barbeque. So we sat round the table over cups of tea and talked until conversation slowly ran out and we retired to our rooms. We are glad we stayed that night with her. It was a lovely, old house; a former ship's captain's I think from the sailing ship era. Like all old houses it was full of atmosphere and memories and it creaked in places as the old building cooled down during the night.

As I lay awake looking up at the ceiling I wondered what Hilary was thinking. Was she asleep? I doubted it but at least she knew she had two friends just a wall's thickness away if she needed us – a much more comforting thought than an empty house.

After breakfast the next morning neighbours and other friends began calling. Hilary was kept very busy so we quietly took our leave, promising we would stay on in Cornwall until the funeral, which we did.

It was more than a week before the funeral was held because of the autopsy which showed that Derrick had an over-enlarged heart. I presume from that that this must involve more than the usual strain on the heart's function but as there was no way of diagnosing this without open chest surgery no-one was aware of it. It is possible that the late afternoon swim in a cold sea might have been the cause. If that was the case at least he was on his favourite beach when the attack occurred. If it had happened in the water his body might not have been recovered for days and possibly weeks as the Cornish coast has many treacherous currents and tides.

The funeral wasn't the sad occasion I expected. The weather was glorious and Derrick was buried in the grounds of a church, which could have graced any tourist calendar depicting churches of old England. The church was packed

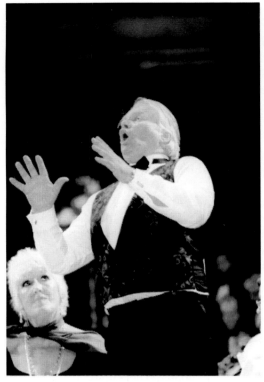

Derrick Phoenix's last concert
for us
with
Maureen McCaulay
awaiting her turn

and everywhere I looked I recognised singers and musicians, most of them from Duchy Opera where Derrick had been a principal soloist.

Ben Luxon spoke the words "The Measure of a Man" in his rich, Cornish voice and Suzanne, accompanied by Anthony on the piano, sang "Remember Me" from Dido and Anaeus. It was a haunting, beautiful song and I don't know how Suzanne managed it without breaking down but she did. There wasn't a dry eye in the congregation afterwards. Members of the Truro Brass Band and the Duchy Choir added their tribute by playing and singing him into and out of the church. Derrick certainly had a great send off, one which I'm sure he would have appreciated and probably did if there is any retention of the spirit after death.

His spirit lived on and Derrick was to be remembers at our 9th Last Night of the Proms in October, which was not far away. I devoted a full page of the souvenir programme as a tribute to him, Ben gave a spoken tribute on stage at the beginning of the evening followed by Suzanne's rendering of "Remember Me" but this time with the choirs and full orchestra. His wife, Hilary, was there as our guest and discovered that night just how much he had meant to us all.

Chapter 23
Tom Allen Joins the Team

As things turned out and such is the way of life as we lost someone special we also gained someone who was also special and it all began on the platform for London-bound travellers at Newcastle Central Station in January 1995. Ben had been performing in a New Year's Eve concert with Northern Sinfonia at the City Hall and, of course, he resided with us. On the morning after the concert, we drove him to the station to catch his train to London. Waiting for the same train was Thomas Allen who, it turned out, had performed on the same night at Durham Cathedral. This chance meeting on a railway platform was to add another touch of magic to our Proms. Ben re-introduced us to Tom because it was many years ago that we had met him and I'm sure he couldn't remember us. However, as soon as Ben mentioned our involvement the North East Proms, Tom immediately said, "I've heard of your "Geordie Prom" and the work you have been doing for cancer research". The conversation went on from there and we couldn't miss an opportunity like that and taking the "bull by the horns" I asked him if he would sing for us one day given the time and opportunity. His reaction was exactly the same as Ben's had been when we approached him about the first concert in 1990, an emphatic "Yes".

We just had time to exchange addresses and telephone numbers when the train pulled in. As they boarded the train, Ben turned and whispered, "Don't worry, Tom's as good as his words and I'll have a chat with him about it on the train".

And that was how Tom Allen came to join the "Team" but it took three years before he could have his debut with us in 1998.

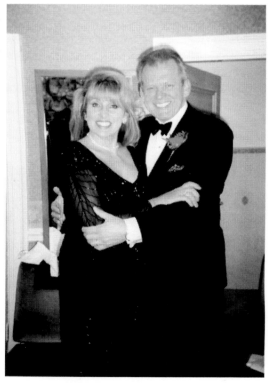

Tom and Janice
waiting to go on stage

One Lump or Two

This had involved a number of letters and phone calls before Tom would safely commit himself, as he was in such great demand worldwide – but it was worth the long wait. We hoped that if Tom could sing for us on a regular annual arrangement, he would be a worthy successor to Ben Luxon, whose serious hearing problems were slowly bringing his singing career to a premature end.

Tom hadn't committed himself at once but he said he was hoping to appear at a concert with Northern Sinfonia on the Friday evening before our Proms concert. It was to be held at Seaham in County Durham, Tom's birthplace and it meant a great deal to him to be there. If this came off he would be happy to stay on an extra couple of days and make a guest appearance for us. It did come off and he was able to appear much to our delight and the many hundreds of fans he had in the North East.

Without any disrespect to any of our other performers, Tom's appearance that night was a great boost to the whole kudos of the Proms. After eight years of unflagging support from the audiences, a new face, especially one so famous and from the North, was probably what was needed if it was to continue like that for a few more years.

Tom's timely arrival also helped to fill the gap left by the tragic death of Derrick Phoenix.

Much of this was caught or mentioned in the final stages of the second television programme which had slowly taken shape right up to the night of the concert. When it was completed it was entitled "George and the Dragon" (Rosalynde still wonders who the dragon was, her or the cancer!). Just before Christmas we made our second half hour appearance on the television channel BBC2. It was televised all over the North East and aroused as much interest and praise as it's predecessor in 1992.

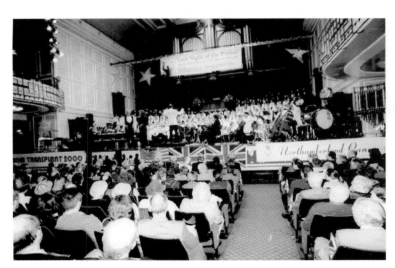

Another full house at the Proms 1999

Chapter 24
A Scottish Holiday and Another Strange Bug

So far 1998 seems to have been a year of holidays, concerts and hospital treatments. Excitement and fun interspersed with the tragedy and heartache and in the last months leading up to Tom Allen's debut it was to happen again. This time it was in the far North West coast of Scotland at a place called Laide; a place I'd never heard of but I'm glad it came our way. This happened because of our friendship with Ian and Jean MacMillan. I first met them on one of the hospital ski weeks in France and spent some time with them improving their skiing. Ian was a Director of Northumbrian Water, one of the newly privatised Water Boards. He not only bought one of my books on that holiday, which greatly interested him, and its story prompted him to ask for more details about how we organised and financed our concerts.

To cut a long story short, Ian was instrumental in involving his company on a guaranteed three years of sponsorship and I'm delighted to say that after completion of those years Northumbrian Water still plays an important role in funding our concerts.

As we came to know Ian and Jean better, and coincidentally Jean was a radiographer at the General so knew well enough what I'd been through, they told us about their crofter's cottage at Laide, which lies between Gairloch and Ullapool. We told them about our cottage in the Cheviots and the idea of using each other's for the occasional holiday was suggested.

As a result we spent a fascinating week there in September 1998 with Marc, Roxanne and Russell. It was a beautiful, lonely place with striking scenery and the cottage looked out to sea where, across the bay, we could see a large barren island rearing out of the water. It was the infamous island of Gruinard, which was used during the 2nd World War for a ghastly experiment in germ warfare. The British, knowing full well that the Germans were experimenting with bombs which spread lethal germs, had to find out if it was possible for germs to survive a bomb blast. This island was chosen and live sheep were deposited on it to test the effects of the blast. The results were terrifying. The germ, which was chosen was anthrax, a deadly killer and it survived the blast killing all the sheep. Unfortunately, the odd body or two somehow fell into the sea and drifted to the mainland causing great distress and panic.

All the sheep had to be burned and the whole island had to be sprayed by people wearing special suits. The island was declared completely out of bounds and I believe it will take hundreds of years before it can be inhabited in any way.

It stood now as a reminder of the stupidity of man and every time I looked at it all I could think of was that poison and death was there in contrast to the beauty which was surrounding it.

It did not spoil the holiday but something else did for me, only me I'm pleased to say. I developed awful stomach pains and spent lengthy times in the toilet. It wasn't something I contracted there, I felt the stirrings a few days before we set off but I just thought I'd eaten something that disagreed with me and it would soon pass. It didn't and also began to affect my appetite and naturally I began to think the worst as I usually do.

I managed to suffer quietly on my own without spoiling things for the rest, who were having a "whale of a time". When we finally reached home though the first thing I did was to tell Rosalynde and the second thing was to contact the RVI and ask for help.

It came from the very doctor who had looked after me throughout the four courses of Rituximab earlier that year, Phil Mounter, one of Steve Proctor's team. He put me through several tests, some more pleasant than others, need I say more. All modesty has to disappear when bowel and intestinal problems strike you down! Finally one of the tests showed that I had thrush in the bowels, of all places. I knew that thrush appeared in other private parts of the body but not in the bowels. Fortunately, after a course of appropriate drugs it cleared up and I recovered fully. I was also very relieved that it was not caused by a return of the lymphoma.

After those weeks of extreme discomfort everything else seemed a pleasure and I tackled the forthcoming concert with more gusto than usual.

Tom Allen lived up to his word and reputation and fitted into this evening as though it was the most natural thing in the world. Knowing Ben, Janice and Northern Sinfonia already was a great help and in the dressing room, it was more like a family reunion than a gathering of professional singers.

When it was all over and we had taken them for the customary, thank you dinner at the Mandarin Restaurant, Tom told us that he had sung on many great occasions all over the world but it was hard for him to remember one of them which could quite match the incredible atmosphere and reception he had experienced and received that night. His very words were "I wish I could bottle the atmosphere which was created tonight and take it with me wherever I go – it was unforgettable".

It was for us too and we knew without doubt that having Tom's support would help to keep things going, certainly for a few more years.

The rest of 1998 was so peaceful and without any further unpleasantries that it seemed an anti-climax to the rest of that turbulent year. Our son, Marc, as I mentioned previously, was having a turbulent year too, his firm in Edinburgh had gone into receivership. He was out of work but what we found out later was the firm owed him several months salary and it looked extremely likely that he would never receive a penny of it. We had been sending him money to help him through the crisis but it was not until later when he finally told us.

Roxanne was fairing better and she and Russell had found and bought a very pleasant stone built, end terrace house in Westerhope, of all places, near our home. We were delighted, of course, and after the usual house buying delays and moving problems, they were now comfortably settled in their first, real home together.

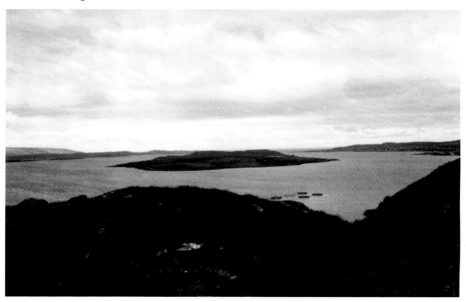

Gruinard Island near Laide

Chapter 25
The End of an Era

1999 should have been a great year; the last of the years with 19 attached to the front and 62 of them had so far covered all my life. Mathematically it wasn't the end of the Millennium as most people seemed to think but everyone was looking at it that way. For me the end of it was nearly my end too!

I talked to Rosalynde at length about the importance of this year and we made our plans; we decided that if we didn't celebrate everything in 1999 it would be a "damp squid" by next year. It was also our 10th anniversary since the first concert in 1990 so we had something extra special, and on a more personal basis, to celebrate. On top of that and with a bit of luck, we would be able to announce that we had reached the target of £500,000, which we had set for that all important decade.

Running alongside this was our son, Marc's, final step into the "real" world of business and employment. I write "real" because he'd had a few failed attempts, not all his fault I must add, but the bonus was that each step seemed to lead him to something better and I could see him grow in stature and maturity.

I also saw the same thing happening to my daughter, Roxanne, who was in the middle of a very steady relationship with a young man called Russell, who we welcomed into the family with open arms. Roxanne, too, had struggled within the employment trap but was also emerging into a new and brighter light. She was working part-time at the Ministry of Agriculture as an Administrative Officer with the Intervention Board but had also followed in Rosalynde's footsteps and studied reflexology for a year at the Newcastle College gaining her qualifications too. She was now helping Rosalynde with her clients and building up a reputation in her own right. I'm very proud of both of them, Marc and Roxanne. They are very different; Marc looks and has a similar personality to Rosalynde – though sadly not her patience. Roxanne ("bossy boots") has taken after me and if she can control her patience there are one or two canny little characteristics from her old dad, which will see her through. She is a wizard with money, Marc is also a wizard with it, but sometimes he has found the art of making it disappear but not bringing it back – he will though, it just takes time. Both of them, like many young people of their generation, have come through really bad, confidence sapping times of unemployment and have survived.

Marc had shone in the academic world during the last two years with a B.Sc. Hons. Degree at Newcastle University and then a M.Sc. at Napier College, Edinburgh. After a couple of redundancy experiences in Edinburgh, he realised he had to go to London for a decent job, money and most importantly experience.

He now works in the world of computers, desk top publishing, the internet etc. and London was the place for any up and coming young graduate in that field. January 1999 was the new beginning for him and he left to take up a Desk Top Publicity Consultant's post with the Stationery Office in London. It was a golden opportunity with a good salary, great prospects and absolute security if he worked hard. Given the time, the opportunity was there for him to grasp, and there was also a whole new ball game out there for him.

It meant giving up Edinburgh for a while; he had grown very fond of it there as a student and stayed on afterwards but Edinburgh does not yet have the same opportunities as London. It also meant leaving his partner, Catherine, a French girl he had met during one of his jobs after University. They, like Roxanne and Russell, were in the middle of a very steady relationship. She, a translator (French into English and vice versa) was self-employed and doing very well although she had to remain in Edinburgh. This proved to be very costly for the pair of them but they were young, in love so what else matters!

Threading along through all this was the beginning of an unease I had that something unaccountable was not right within me. It was slowly coming up to a year since my last successful treatment plus the new drug (Rituximab) which I'd had but the first year always seemed the big hurdle. I always regularly checked myself and I always kept my fingers mentally crossed till I was satisfied I couldn't find anything but something began niggling away at my confidence. I had also built up my hopes that this new drug just might be the big hope I'd been waiting for and the answer to my prayers

I had my usual check ups and blood tests at the RVI but nothing positive showed up. My appetite, however, was not what it should be and suddenly I began to experience strange fluttering feelings in the heart area of my chest. I also found I was out of breath going up the stairs or on the hilly parts of the golf course – most unusual for me.

I expressed my concern to Steve Proctor on one of my visits and he checked my heart thoroughly but could find nothing amiss. He thought, as he had mentioned on previous occasions that I was prone to stress reactions being a "hyperactive sort of guy" as he put it. I felt like telling him that running a charity had, in fact, become one of the most stressful parts of my life and Rosalynde's too for that matter. We both enjoyed it most of the time and had had some wonderful times, meeting fantastic people and doing some good as we went along. Hard to complain about that, really!

Steve, being as thorough as ever, decided to check the heart function out properly and arranged for me to see a specialist at the RVI, a Dr Skinner. She was very nice, following in the tradition of all the other medics I've dealt with and I was put through every test possible as far as I could tell – everything was fine. So what was wrong! Steve put me on a short dose of steroids to boost my appetite which did the trick but the fluttering and breathlessness still persisted and worst of all my golf began to suffer!

Anyone reading my first book would see that fell walking in the Cheviots and skiing abroad had been my forte during those early years of fighting cancer. Golf was there too but it played a more minor role.

Ten years on, both Rosalynde and I had suffered several skiing injuries, which made us realise we were not getting any younger; the recovery time afterwards was becoming longer and even I was beginning to look at some of the black runs with some trepidation. The winter snows hadn't been as good as in previous years and as I'd skied and taught skiing since the seventies I began to think of calling it a day. Although I hadn't tired of walking in the Cheviots there was hardly a mile around the northern and eastern area, where we had our cottage, which I hadn't walked and on more than one occasion.

My very dear walking partner, Emily Watson, was slowly and majestically approaching 70. I write "majestically" because she had gone through major heart surgery and she was now suffering from Parkinson's disease – but what a fighter and what a spirit! This had sadly slowed her lifestyle down but she was as active in many other ways. We still spent hours together keeping our two cottages and gardens in good repair and looking tidy and we made a great grass-cutting team. We still walked but I cut the distance I walked and heights climbed even more much to Rosalynde's satisfaction. We still, however, managed some very lovely walks in what I still call "Gods' gift to the Northumbrians" and, of which, I am proud to be one; a Northumbrian I mean, not a gift from God!

It was golf which had slowly but inevitably crept in to take their places and although I had played the game reasonably well over a large number of years it had never replaced my other real interests.

Now I loved it and was slowly but surely building the same enjoyment of the game for Rosalynde – once a teacher always a teacher! I have never achieved anything but enjoyment and satisfaction, oh yes, and much frustration, from this wonderful, innocently – easy looking game. I did, however, have one brief moment of glory. I scored a hole in one in a bonafide competition at my favourite golf course, the Hirsel Golf Club at Coldstream.

This brilliant golfing episode should have been in my first book but in the rather dramatic cuts, which took place during the editing process, it was one of the cuts. It was something I regretted very much afterwards because not only was it my brief moment of glory but it was a very, very funny and absolutely true golfing story. Some of my golfing friends will probably say that I have really written my second book just to make sure the world knows about my hole in one.

It happened like this ....

Chapter 26
My Hole in One at the Hirsel Golf Club, Berwickshire

Way back in 1976 we rented a one-storeyed farm cottage at Tithe Farm about four miles further North from our existing cottage at Kypie Farm. The children were very young and we spent as much time as possible with them at this idyllic little spot near the Scottish border. We had a family country membership at the 9 hole golf course called the Hirsel Golf Club, which was laid out on part of Sir Alec Douglas Home's estate near Coldstream.

Our next door neighbours at this cottage were Bernard and Denise Baxter and their exuberant, fun-loving sons Tony, Graham and Ben, all of whom played golf and were also members at the Hirsel. Bernard was Headmaster and I was his Youth and Community Deputy Headmaster and we worked at Longbenton High School, at that time. He had shown an interest in our cottage when he took up his post in 1970 and I had introduced him to the farmer, who had subsequently rented the next door cottage to him when it became vacant.

Both families were at Tithe Hill for the weekend and it was mid September. Bernard asked me if I would like to enter the monthly medal with him on the Saturday. If we played together, he and I could mark each other's card. Rosalynde and Denise joined us as a foursome but not in the competition. We dropped all the kids off in Coldstream where they wanted to wander around the shops after which they said they would walk to the golf course and join us there.

The weather was quite good and we made an early start. I was a little nervous, I am not a good competitive player, I tend to worry about my shots and this usually leads to erratic play. However, that morning started well and by the time I reached the 7th hole my score was reasonably impressive. The 7th is an interesting, short hole played from high ground, over a stream and on to a wide green; about 105 yards altogether and usually played with a wedge or a 9 iron, depending on the wind. Bernard had won the last hole making it his honour and his shot landed between the stream and the green. I teed my ball up and looked down towards the flag to gauge the wind's direction and strength from it. I noticed Marc, Roxanne and Bernard's boys all sitting on the gate near the green where the Hirsel Road ran alongside the course. Immediately I felt tension creeping in as I realised I had an audience. I tried to blot out all thoughts of the ball landing ignominiously in the stream and kept my head down as I swung at the ball. It felt right and I looked up in time to see it soar high over the stream and land just inside the near edge of the green in line with the pin. What happened next was a joy to see, the ball bounced twice before settling into a slow rolling

My "infamous" hole in one scorecard!

HIRSEL GOLF CLUB

COLDSTREAM BERWICKSHIRE.

Name... George Walker

Date... 11 Sep 76... Competition... Medal

Holes	Yards	Par	Stroke Hole	Score	Hole	Yards	Par	Stroke Hole	Score
1	304	4	11	6	10	304	4	12	5
2	283	4	13	5	11	283	4	14	5
3	235	4	15	4	12	235	3	16	4
4	316	4	7	4	13	316	4	8	4
5	345	4	5	6	14	345	4	4	5
6	414	4	3	5	15	414	4	2	4
7	103	3	17	1	16	103	3	18	4
8	337	3	9	6	17	337	4	10	5
9	491	5	1	6	18	491	5	6	8
	2828	35		43		2828	35	In	44
						2828	35	Out	43

S.S.S. 67
Par 70

Marker's Signature — fW.) Baxter

Player's Signature — GWalker

	5656	Total	87
		Handicap	20
		Nett	67

How & Blackhall, Printers, Berwick.

pace as it headed towards the hole. I held my breath then yelled out in delight as the ball vanished into the hole. Out of the corner of my eye I could see Marc and the rest of the youngsters leaping off the gate and waving madly at me. By this time my No. 9 iron had gone hurtling into the air as I flung it skywards in celebration. Bernard, Denise and Rosalynde gathered around me and were congratulating me on my shot. I retrieved my iron, walked down the hill and crossed the small footbridge to meet my young and enthusiastic admirers. If I ever had to pick an event in a lifetime of my sporting activities, it would be that short moment in time on a Scottish golf course in full view of my family. Sadly, I haven't done anything else since to brook such a reward.

The game continued and my card, much improved by a 1 written on it, had the makings of a winner. By the time I reached the 18th tee which is also the 9th, however, I became nervous because if there was ever a hole to blow it, this was the one. It was a long par 5 with a narrow fairway bounded on one side by a road, which was out of bounds. I didn't make a good connection and watched glumly as my first ball sliced away and seemed to land just over the fence between the semi rough and the road. I had to place another ball on the tee and try again just in case it was out of bounds. I made absolutely sure this time as the ball flew over the fence, the road and into a field full of sheep. A third ball had to be placed on the tee making it six strokes so far and I felt suicidal. My partners had fallen silent and I could almost feel their concern for my predicament. It was a cautious strike this time but the ball made it to the fairway and I breathed a sigh of relief. "It's going to be a hell of a job to complete this hole in under 10", I grimly though as I walked along the fence in the hope that my first ball might still be in bounds and playable. Someone up there must have loved me that day because when I reached the spot where it had disappeared, there it was within bounds and, although not in the best of spots, still playable. I shouted to Bernard that I'd found it and would he pick up my third ball, which was near his on the fairway. I took a lofted club out of my bag and managed to punch the ball out of the semi rough grass on to the fairway. It was a test of nerves after that and I messed it up again by 3 putting and finally managed to complete what was almost a disaster with an 8 which brought my total to 87. Allowing for my handicap of 20 I netted a 67 for a much reduced but still reasonable chance of winning the competition.

Back at the clubhouse Bernard signed my card, which I still have to this day, and I handed it to the secretary. He looked at it and said immediately, "So, you're the fellow who got a hole in one, well your card looks a possible winner and I've got some even better news for you. Sir Alec Douglas Home is president of the club and he always presents a cheque for £15.00 to anyone who gets a hole in one in a club competition. The Scottish Sunday Post also gives a brand new putter to a bone fide "hole in one" scorer providing it's in a competition and on a Scottish golf course. Well done laddie".

We went into the bar to celebrate. Word had obviously got around about my success and, in the old tradition, I stood drinks for everyone present. I had to borrow some money from Bernard as there were quite a few people present. The round came to nearly £18.00. A costly business in those days but I didn't care – the honour of the moment and rewards yet to come made up for my pecuniary embarrassment.

As we had been early starters, it would be a long wait to find out if I had won the competition. It was well after lunchtime anyway so Bernard suggested we return to the farm, have lunch then fill in the rest of the afternoon with a game of bridge. We could return to the club for an early evening drink and find out how we'd got on. It seemed a good idea so we packed the children into the cars and headed back into England.

After a hastily prepared lunch, the youngsters settled down to watch a film on our tiny black and white portable television while we became engrossed in a game of bridge. This was livened up with occasional glasses of Bernard's and

Rosalynde's potent home brews.

The room grew darker as the afternoon wore on and I looked out of the window to see the weather changing rapidly as dark heavy rain clouds loomed over us. Even the deceptive warmth of alcohol couldn't prevent a slight chill creeping into the room, so I said I would light the fire. I went outside to the coalhouse and found the stick box empty. I took the axe in one hand and a log of wood in the other and began rhythmically chopping the log into smaller pieces. Each sweep of the axe brought its vicious looking blade nearer and nearer to the hand holding of the log. I'm convinced that what happened next was a combination of the confident mood I was in and too much celebratory alcohol. I became fascinated with the arc of the swinging axe and the diminishing log I was holding. Next second the fascination vanished as, suddenly, I found my hand transfixed to the log and blood spurting out of the wound where the sharp corner of the axe had pierced my hand before embedding itself into the wood. Surprisingly there wasn't any immediate pain, just a cold numbness within the injured hand. I moaned with the shock and stood up without thinking. The axe, my hand and the log came up as one with me and I wasn't holding the log. I staggered to the door and realised I couldn't open it so literally, using my head, I banged it as hard as I could on the door. Pain was overcoming the numbness in my hand by now and my head wasn't feeling too good either with the continuous banging! Eventually it opened and Rosalynde peered into the gloom wondering why I couldn't open the door myself. She soon found out as I sheepishly held out my hand still pinned to the log by the axe.

She helped me inside and that was the end of the bridge game. It is very difficult holding 13 cards with an axe through your hand! Seriously though, it was quite a shock and everyone realised it could be very serious. The axe was gently released from my hand and the block of wood and my bloodied hand was quickly washed and bandaged. As weekends are not the best of times to find a doctor the decision was made to take me to the Coldstream Cottage Hospital, which ironically, is next to the golf course and it has an accident and emergency ward. The nurse in charge wasn't very sympathetic when she found out how and what I'd done.

"Sit over there, laddie, I'll deal with you in a moment. I've got more important things to do – I've got a lassie expecting twins in the next room" was her welcome in the lovely soft burr of the Scottish Borders. Her bark was worse than her bite though, because she was soon back and bustling around me.

"Have ye had a tetanus injection in recent years?"

I said no and she made me whip my trousers down and stuck a needle in my backside without batting an eyelid. I then saw the doctor, who turned out to be a golfer and was a little more sympathetic. He checked my hand thoroughly and said I had been extremely lucky the corner of the blade had gone through the hand without damaging the bone or cutting the tendons. Both sides just needed stitching. After this was done the nurse bandaged the hand and put it in a sling.

"No more golf for a few weeks", was her parting advice as I left the hospital "and report to your own doctor to have the stitches removed by the end of the week".

Outside, in more pain than when I'd gone in, we checked the time and wondered what to do next. It was decided that rather than go back to the cottage then return for the evening and competition results, we would just call at the clubhouse and see how I'd fared. It made sense as we were so close to the place but deep down I wasn't looking forward to entering the clubhouse looking like the walking wounded from a war film; I would have to explain my predicament to one and all.

We did just that and everyone was sympathetic in between a few leg-pulling comments. Then came the bombshells.............

The club secretary approached us and I repeated my story for about the third time. He then said, "Well I've got some more bad news for you. You didn't win, you were second. Actually you tied with someone else and if that happens we always take the second nine scores and he beat you by one". I thought, "That was that bloody 18th hole" and said, "Well, at least second is some consolation". "Sorry", said the secretary, "but I understand you are just a country member", I waited expectantly, "and unfortunately a club ruling is that country members can take part in competitions but not win them unless they have a handicap given by this club". I couldn't argue with that as my handicap was based on the club at Westerhope where I lived. Still, there was £15.00 and a putter to come, they couldn't take that away from me. "Oh yes" the secretary went on, "I've checked on your hole in one and Sir Alec only gives the £15.00 once every year and someone had a hole in one in the August competition. Tough luck, old chap". I didn't feel like asking about the putter, I seemed to know I wouldn't get it but things couldn't get that bad so I plucked up courage and said, "What about the Sunday Post prize"? "I've checked up on that too and", wait for it, "The Sunday Post offer is a monthly one and runs through the summer season which expired on 31 August.

I left the clubhouse that night a broken man in mind and body!

Like all defeated champions, I bounced back and my challenge has since been to win a competition and to break 80 gross in a golf round. I've had an 81 and come close to it several times but I always seem to botch it at the end when I'm almost there. I've finally had an 80 this summer but the elusive 79 is still out there.

Chapter 27
A Year of Preparation and Celebration

I mentioned earlier that 1999 was the climax for our £500,000 target special and we needed to produce something really worthy to celebrate the 10 years it took and combine it with the Millennium celebrations.

Golf and the strange chest murmers were pushed to one side as Rosalyne and I became embroiled in our plans for this but my unease was always there. I also had losses of appetite, which in my limited knowledge is always a cause for concern and I wonder, even now, why this wasn't looked into more closely. Blood tests didn't show anything out of the ordinary, which I had always been told was a good sign and I was given the occasional prescription for steroids, which certainly boosted the appetite but made me even more hyperactive than I usually am. Looking back I feel quite strongly that the appetite should have been looked at more closely and not just hidden by steroids. The real problem is that only a CT scan or other internal examinations can really identify anything properly and there is a limit to the number of scans you can have. As far as the steroids were concerned, Rosalynde woke up one morning to the sound of hammering in my garden shed. It was 5.30 am and I was working on some restoration work of a chair that I'd picked up very cheaply at a bric and brac shop. It was a lovely sunny morning and I'd woken up full of energy and enthusiasm. I won't describe what she said to me.

Our Millennium and Anniversary celebrations turned into three concerts and spread over the year. We started with Suzanne Manuell's Annual Concert at the Newcastle Civic Centre for which we needed a very special guest to join her and we were fortunate indeed to acquire the services of Bradley Creswick, who is not only the leader of the Northern Sinfonia but a violin soloist in his own right with a high national as well as local profile.

He had performed several solo pieces at our proms, which left us in no doubt as to his calibre and popularity. We were delighted when he accepted our invitation and confirmed all the arrangements.

The "Last Night" needed more thought and preparation because of its sheer size and previous success. It had to be exceptional and we looked through all the previous nine programmes for inspiration and finally decided we would produce a concert of highlights from those programmes but adding something new at the same time.

Ben Luxon, Janice Cairns and Suzanne Manuell all confirmed they could sing again for us on the date we had selected and we waited, with fingers crossed, for Tom Allen, who is now Sir Thomas Allen after being knighted by the Queen in her 1999 Birthday Honours List – a well-deserved honour, too. Tom is younger than Ben and between them they commanded all the great operatic baritone roles in all the opera houses of note in Britain, Europe and America. Ben's career had begun to peak, accelerated by his severe deafness, whilst Tom still had those additional years to come.

Ben's initial presence in 1990 turned the Proms concert into what it became, a prestigious event, which gathered a huge following every year thereafter. Ben continues helping us with the Proms and has not missed singing in any of them since they began. We were thrilled that he would be there at the 10th even though it might be his last. During our last three years he had withdrawn from operatic arias and singing in the choral pieces simply because he couldn't hear himself pitch the notes anymore. His voice was as good as ever but if you hit the wrong note with his booming baritone voice everyone in the audience would know it. I asked him how he managed and he just said "I have to sing the notes from memory and I hope I get them right". The stress, too, became more obvious as the concerts approached; he wasn't enjoying his music anymore and we felt very guilty that we still clung to him for his expertise and charisma. Ben isn't much taller than me (I'm 5'8") but he has a bulkier frame. He always looks tall and imposing on stage and television and people are very surprised when they meet him. He has that extra star quality, which switches on like a light when he appears in front of an audience. Our audiences love him and always give him a great reception. They are all aware of his predicament as we've never tried to hide his hearing disability and his charisma always carries him through any performance he does.

When Tom Allen finally rang to say he could sing for us again, I think Ben was as relieved as we were. It took the pressure off Ben and he could relax more and enjoy the singing.

This leads me on to the third and final concert of the Millennium. Two things I wanted to do most of all and the first was to have something for Ben to perform, which I knew he could do well and his hearing wouldn't cause him stress or embarrassment. I had a feeling this concert would be his last so I wanted him to go out with a bang. The other thing was to bring as many of the performers together who had sang or played for us over the 10 years. I knew it would be impossible for them all to come because of their other engagements but I had to try. We decided to call it a "Special Millennium Concert Party Night" and the emphasis would be on party rather than concert. I also decided to include the whole of the Luxon family because of their involvement in the 10 years and our publicity emphasised the appearance of the "Von Luxon" family rather like the Von Trapps of "Sound of Music" fame. The Luxons are a very musically talented family. Sheila, Ben's wife, has been a principal soprano with Benjamin Britten's English Opera group and they had met performing together in one of the company's operas. She had stepped in during the first two of our Proms after Janice Cairns had to pull out following a dreadful accident to her spine whilst performing in Tosca at the London Coliseum. Even when Janice

One Lump or Two

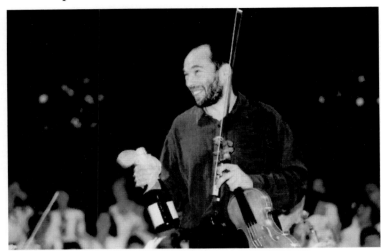

*Suzanne
&
Anthony's
special guest,
Bradley
Creswick*

finally joined us Sheila sang with her in a couple more of the Proms and was always very popular. Sheila and Ben had sadly separated as I mentioned earlier but it was good to see them meet again as friends. Rachel, their daughter, was following in mum's footsteps after discovering she had a beautiful soprano voice. She had studied for a degree in music and had then continued her singing studies at the Glasgow Royal Academy of Music and Drama. She is currently studying opera at the Manchester College of Music and Drama and is slowly making a name for herself. Daniel has discovered, unfortunately rather late in life, that he has a fine tenor voice, his rendering of "Nessum Dorma", is very accomplished, top notes and all. Jonathan has a gentle baritone voice on the classical side but his real love is the guitar and modern music so I had a feeling he would probably not become involved.

The only thing left to do before going ahead with all the complicated arrangements was to see who could come and help us celebrate and amazingly only Tom Allen and Bradley couldn't; Tom was performing in an opera somewhere in Europe and Bradley was on a tour of Germany with Northern Sinfonia. It was disappointing of course but good fortune smiled on us and Rachel's boyfriend, James Cleverton, who had studied with her at Glasgow had a fine operatic bass-baritone voice and offered his services. I had also telephoned the young and up and coming concert violinist, Sian Philipps, who had already performed for us on two occasions to much acclaim. Sian was a graduate of the Guildhall School of Music and the Yehudi Menuhin School for Violinists and was a wonderful solo performer. She accepted our invitation immediately and our cast was complete. But before that we had to oversee the 10th Anniversary Last Night – the most important of them all – a grand celebration of 10 years, £500,000.00 raised for cancer research and patient care.

Chapter 28
The Tenth "Proms"

What a night, very little sleep, lists of things running backwards and forwards in my mind. Much needed rehearsal, which had been cancelled by Northern Sinfonia on Friday had added more pressure to everyone but there was nothing we could do about it. Everyone would have to rehearse together for the first time during the Saturday afternoon schedule. Thank goodness there wasn't a Newcastle United home game at the same time. Access through the "toon", as Newcastle is affectionately known, is almost impossible on match days.

After breakfast I set off first as usual with a car full of "props" for the City Hall. Some of my stalwart helpers were already there and raring to go. My first major problem sprang at me like a cold shower when Alan Young told me they were going to be short of paper bags for the "Geordie Cannons" during the 1812 Overture. I had ordered 10,000 from Kimberly Clark, one of our benefactors, but the delivery note showed 2,500. I couldn't believe it as there seemed more than enough when I'd loaded the car and I'd even left a huge pile back home in the garage. I telephoned Rosalynde, who was on the "emergency line" back home and she tracked down Edwin Mutton, Kimberly Clark's contact man, and she came back with the news that I should wear my spectacles when checking delivery notes. There had been 25,000 paper bags delivered not 2,500! Rosalynde calculated that I must have over 15,000 spare bags in the garage! The bags were very important – what a relief.

I had suggested to Kimberly Clark via Edwin that as well as printing the firm's logo on the bags that they printed an appropriate message and he asked me to send him a draft. I did and it went like this:-

Unfold bag
Blow it up
Wait for signal from Conductor
Burst bag
Prepare next one

It looked good on the finished product and I'm sure the audience would appreciate the joke.

With that major problem out of the way, the day proceeded well and by lunchtime the Hall was transformed and ready for the evening. The new banners showing the 10 company sponsors looked very striking hanging above the stage.

The programmes arrived fresh from the printers and looked immensely impressive. The two John's at Creative Art and Design and Amanda, their very able assistant, had put everything I'd given them into a souvenir booklet of which they could be very proud and it would certainly do the whole show justice when they went on sale that evening and hopefully make us a profit.

One Lump or Two

People began to drift in for rehearsals and I finally had something to eat with Rosalynde and then we started to plan what we were going to say on the stage at the end of the show – always the most difficult part for us.

By having ten shared sponsors and to make sure they all felt included in the plans and action, I had persuaded Steve Proctor to print some "Certificates of Recognition" from his research charity for them and the performers. We had them properly and appropriately framed but not before a friend, Gretta Wilson, inscribed their names individually on each certificate in the most beautifully done calligraphy work I've seen for a while. It took her three whole days and they looked splendid.

These had to be presented – but when? We were under terrific pressure to finish by 10.30 pm. Normal limit is 10 pm but we'd managed to persuade the orchestra, which was bound by strict Union rules, to allow us to go over time on this occasion; within reason of course. We decided to present them at the beginning of the second half when all the fun began.

The last big hurdle was the presentation of gifts to the performers and the "thank you" speeches, which we've traditionally slotted in before the finale of Jerusalem and Auld Lang Syne, in which everyone in the Hall joins in singing. Tonight was more special than usual and I couldn't see how it could be cut down in any way if I was to give justice to everyone, who had been behind us during the 10 years.

I had spent some enjoyable hours during the year looking for individual and very personal gifts to be presented to the conductors and our singing stars. I had decided on paintings because collecting paintings is my hobby and I have a great instinct for finding pictures even though I cannot paint or draw in the slightest.

I was very pleased with what I'd found and the only disappointment to me when we finally presented them on stage was that there wasn't time for them to be opened and shown to the audience, as the gifts were from them too as well as Rosalynde and me. Suffice to say, the recipients told me afterwards that my choices could not have been better or more appropriate.

I have already mentioned earlier in this book that Thomas Allen, the Seaham born (County Durham) baritone had joined our "team" of stars, making his debut in the 9th concert in 1998 with a rendering of Figaro's Aria from the Barber of Seville, which brought the house to its feet shouting for more. He was knighted for his services to music in the Queen's Birthday Honours List in June 1999. So it was now Sir Thomas Allen appearing with Ben, Janice and Suzanne tonight, a proud moment for us and one, which had been taken up by the press. This had given a massive boost to our publicity and of course, for the sponsors. It had taken the form of an eight page colour supplement commemorating the 10th Anniversary, which had been distributed by the Journal throughout the North East and had more than a little to do with us selling every last ticket.

Although we became desperately stretched for time at the end of the evening, the plans fell into shape except at the very end of the speeches. Rosalynde's big moment, after adding a few words of thanks to mine, traditionally arrived when she called for a roll of drums. At this point a couple of orchestra members had the task of tugging two pieces of invisible fishing lines, which were tied to a banner above the orchestra's and choir's heads. This was then supposed to unfurl and show everyone the amount raised with a huge "Thank You" painted below it. This exercise always worked during rehearsals but it had occasionally gone wrong at the critical moments. That night was another critical moment. The musicians tugged, the drums rolled and the audience gasped in sympathy mixed with expectation. I didn't know what to do. Rosalynde looked at me and I mouthed "say the amount over the microphone", which she was just about to do, when a last desperate tug did the trick and the banner unfurled revealed £500,000.00 for all to see. Ten years of effort reaching its climax. Actually, we were a little short of reaching that target after we'd finally totted up all the bills afterwards. It didn't really matter because we still had the millennium concert to come and we would be well over that target by the end of it with weeks to spare.

There is no doubt in my mind and in most other people's too, judging by the newspaper review, the phone calls and the letters which followed on over the next few days, that this 10th Concert had been the very best of them all and in spite of not having the full rehearsal time, a great credit to the performers.

The questions immediately sprang to my mind when the dust had settled was "Is there to be an 11th in the year 2000 and can we out-do this one?" What actually happens and it is pride that makes me mention this, is that we have received similar comments after every Proms concert so far. Each one is the best but each one is better than the one before. Does that make sense? The feeling of pride is not just for myself, it is for everyone involved in making the concerts so successful. Can we maintain this standard is the third question but only time can answer that question.

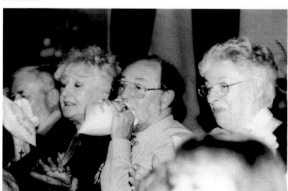

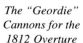

The "Geordie" Cannons for the 1812 Overture

Chapter 29
The Millennium Concert and More Health Problems

Coming near the end of this story is probably the hardest of all my writings and I include the first book in this. "Cancer is Only a Word" had its sad moments but throughout it I always had the feeling that things would eventually turn out in my favour and the final chapter ended on a healthy, high note.

Since then much has happened to erode these thoughts and events of the last few weeks have probably been the hardest of them all apart from that very first week in 1988 when I was told I only had 12 weeks to live. I haven't, however, given up and who knows by the time I finish things may have changed for the better.

The problem is that after nearly 12 years and several recurrences my options are running out every time there is another occurrence. My body is 12 years older, it's had a terrific hammering from chemotherapy and radiotherapy, which says a lot for it, but how long can it stand the constant attacks both from the illness and the treatment. Mentally too I've taken a beating and I find it harder and harder to draw on my reserves of strength and character. Still I'm a "stubborn bastard" as people keep telling me and there is "life in the old dog yet".

This last episode began in November after the Millennium Concert on the 27th. Rosalynde and I were literally exhausted with concert planning and work and we had a large number of people to look after. I had been over-ambitious as usual and the "something special" was almost proving too much for us. The "party" idea had caught the imagination of our public and it was a sell out so that was no problem. It was just the logistics of it all. Our friends had rallied round to accommodate the performers we had no rooms for and they were going to ferry everyone around to rehearsals etc but the arrangements and decisions were mine really as I'd done all the planning so the burden was lying heavily on my shoulders. Without Rosalynde's help and patience throughout this hectic period it would have become a nightmare. She looked after all the catering and boarding arrangements with our friends as well as helping me with other things. This left me to get on with the production itself with all its fiddly, frustrating intricacies.

The evening itself was a great success if not a little long. We had to give our performers a reasonable involvement in the programme. Janice was travelling from Portsmouth, Ben, Suzanne and Anthony from Cornwall, Sheila from Canterbury, Sian from East Sussex and so on, so it had to be worth their while in performance time.

It didn't help matters when I arrived in a rush from home to open up. Fortunately, some of the helpers had already arrived and people were flocking in. I rushed up to the stage with my notes and various bits and pieces while Rosalynde dashed to make sure the catering arrangements were in hand for the buffet meal, which she had arranged for our performers and sponsors after the concert.

I was flapping around on the stage with the microphone and my notes like a one-armed paperhanger when I put my hand in my pocket for something and felt that my bunch of car keys seemed larger than usual. Imagine my horror when I pulled two sets out and instantly recognised Ben's keys, which had been lying ready for him on our dresser at home. They were similar to mine and I must have just picked them up in dashing to get away. Ben was bringing his car in with Suzanne and Anthony and they were now stuck in Westerhope. The concert was due to start in 20 minutes with Ben and Anthony the first to go on.

I panicked, literally panicked, all that careful planning was going to be ruined by a bunch of bloody keys.

Keys and, more recently, spectacles have always been the bane of my life. I have spent hours looking for the damned things.

It even went back to the 1960s. The worst and funniest example of this happened at the end of a very long, hard day and evening at Longbenton High School. I was working in my office in the huge, purpose built Youth and Adult Centre, which I ran and it was just coming up to 10 pm when we closed.

I had a sophisticated tannoy system in my office and could tannoy messages all over the building . At 9.50 pm I, or whoever was on duty, tannoyed a closing down message. I had just done this when one of my staff came in to see me. When he left I looked for my keys on my desk, which had already been "lost" several times that evening. The keys were very important e.g. locking the safe, desk, office and a special key for my office alarm. I couldn't leave until I found them and everyone else was about to depart and it was a very large building to search.

I was so tired and frustrated I burst out in an angry, loud voice. "I've lost my f......g keys again"! Believe me, I don't use that word often, only in extreme circumstances but at those sort of times it seems to say it all! It's a word in very common use now, sadly, but it shocked then.

I sensed rather than heard the building go quiet. I had an observation window in my office, which looked into the large reception area and I glanced at it almost instinctively. Everyone in that area, and there were many, was looking towards my office. Then in a flash it dawned on me - I had left tannoy switched ON and my message had travelled throughout the whole building!

It took me a long time to live that down but strangely enough the "hard lads" in the Youth Section looked at me with greater respect after that!

One Lump or Two

Tonight's keys episode was not quite so amusing and I looked around desperately thinking of how I could get Ben and his company there in time. I visualised Ben looking everywhere for his keys and I knew he would know instinctively that it was something to do with me. I saw Ian Turner, a very good friend of ours, who is also a Trustee of our Charity; he could see I was uptight and came over.

"Anything wrong"? he asked.

"Ian, you'll never believe this but I've come away from home with Ben's car keys leaving him stranded with Anthony and Suzanne".

Ian reacted straightaway, took Ben's keys and dashed off to Westerhope in his car. I returned to the stage and began to frantically plan a stalling exercise until Ben and Anthony could make their appearances. That wasn't easy, people had been coming in since 6 o'clock, the concert was due to start at 6.45 pm, which had now arrived. They were sitting expectantly. I felt over 500 pairs of eyes looking at me. With a last frantic look at the hall door I began to ad lib. The audience roared with delight when I told them I'd stranded Ben, Suzanne and Anthony so that was a good start – my reputation had already gone before me. Encouraged by this I started telling a couple of jokes which also went down well and as I began searching for another I saw Ben and Anthony come through the door in the nick of time.

We were running 15 minutes late but the evening sped past – and I think we gave everyone their money's worth by the end of it. Ben did his dramatisation of Lord Tennyson's epic story poem "Enoch Arden" with Anthony accompanying him on the piano in true Victorian style. They were both in period costume and the stage was done up with the appropriate period furniture too.

Ben also masterminded the second half as Master of Ceremonies and the audience showed its appreciation at the end of it in their North East fashion. Once again it had all been worth it and our funds were richer by £6,000.00.

A few days later Rosalynde and I came down with what we thought was the dreaded flu bug. Rosalynde eventually recovered but I didn't and this leads on to the sequence, which now begins to unfold.

The bug seemed to attack my chest and I thought I was heading for bronchitis. I became worse and, fortunately, it coincided with a visit to the RVI for a check up with Steve Proctor. It turned out he was away and his senior registrar, Jim Cavet, was taking the clinic. I'd been seen by Jim on an earlier occasion and he knew about the difficulties I'd had with the chest murmurs and breathing. Rosalynde came with me and when we saw Jim I could see he knew something was wrong. He sent me straight down for an x-ray, which I returned to him, and he showed us the right lung was filling up with fluid. He then told me the only way to find out what was causing the fluid was to take a sample by needle, which had to be done with local anaesthetic.

It had to be done so I braced myself – I've had so many needles stuck in me over the years that I balk every time I have to face a needle now. Jim made a professional job of it and it wasn't as bad as I expected. The fluid was sent off for examination and we could only wait for the outcome. Next evening we received a phone call at home from our GP saying the hospital had been in touch and they wanted me in first thing in the morning. Naturally, we slept badly that night thinking the worst and that feeling remained with us until we saw Dr Cavet.

Incredible as it may seem they had found salmonella in the fluid and it was growing and attacking the pleura and lung. Although it was quite a shock I felt a huge surge of relief because of expecting the worst, a recurrence of my old enemy. Salmonella and all the things I'd heard about it I could cope with, the other was a different matter.

I had always thought that salmonella was a virus which attacked the intestines and stomach resulting in very serious sickness and diarrhoea but I found out later that on very rare occasions it lodged in and attacked other parts of the body, in my case my lungs.

At the hospital they immediately put me on a very strong dosage of antibiotics but another x-ray a week later showed only a slight decrease in the amount of fluid and my breathing was not much better. Steve Proctor said he would refer me to a chest specialist. The specialist examined the x-rays and my chest very thoroughly and said, in his opinion, the reason why the salmonella was clinging to its hold was because it had lodged itself in pockets in the wall of the pleura and had built up its own "walls" of resistance to the antibiotics. The only way to solve this was to go into the chest surgically and literally clean them out. He said he could arrange this with a colleague at the Freeman Hospital where chest operations were carried out. We agreed to his going ahead but it turned into a nightmare.

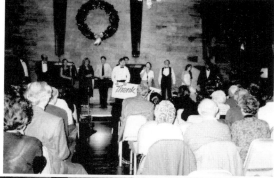

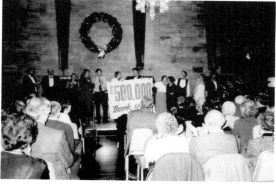

The Millennium Concert "Team" at the Civic Centre - Newcastle when we reached the £500,000 target.

Chapter 30
The Freeman Hospital

The Freeman is a fairly new hospital alongside the older Newcastle hospitals such as the RVI & the General. Heart and lung cases were dealt with at the Freeman. It is situated on the southeast side of Newcastle and looks very modern and very big. It was to play a major role in events that befell me over the Millennium celebrations and the weeks following them.

I was admitted to the RVI on 21st December 99 for tests, x-rays and a line inserted to drain fluid from the pleura, which was severely affecting my breathing. An unbelievable total of over three litres was drained off, no wonder I couldn't breathe! The drain was then removed so that I could return home for Christmas. Our Christmas pattern was the same as in previous years but there was, unfortunately, a cloud of uncertainty hanging over it. It was nice to be home though and Marc came from London to spend it with us. Catherine, his partner, had gone to France to be with her family and they would both meet up with each other again in Edinburgh for the Millennium celebrations. Roxanne arrived, too, and stayed over Christmas Eve and Christmas Day and we had a very enjoyable day, opening presents followed by Christmas dinner and the inevitable drinks and chocolates as we watched the more interesting television programmes in the evening.

Too soon by far, I was back in the RVI and then transferred the next day, the 29th December, by ambulance to the Freeman hospital to prepare for a chest operation to clear the pockets of salmonella poisoning, which had resisted the anti-biotics. I must admit I had no idea it was going to be such major surgery and the chest would need to be opened for the surgeon to go in to find and then clean out the pockets. I had some misguided idea about keyhole surgery. I was soon to be put completely in the picture!

After the nil by mouth procedure and the pre operation injection, I was wheeled into the operating theatre and once again didn't know another thing more until I awoke in the High Dependency Unit, where I spent the next, rather painful 24 hours before being returned to a Ward as they were closing the Unit down over the Millennium weekend. I had my first experience of morphine and it was self injected. This is very clever because it is impossible to overdose even though you appear to self inject too often at times. Only a measured and timed amount goes into the body no matter how many times you press the button. Psychologically though you are sure additional relief from pain is on its way every time you press.

I survived that and was returned to a ward where the morphine injector and saline drip, which had also been connected to me was removed. It was then I really appreciated the help I received from the morphine as the pain returned

132

with a vengeance but I now had to rely on normal painkillers. By then it was actually New Year's Eve and the beginning of the Millennium celebrations. Rosalynde returned again in the evening and we celebrated with patients who also had to stay in during this time. Sadly, it was not much of a celebration and not what we had planned but at least we were together for such an important and historical occasion and that was all that really mattered. Rosalynde was determined that we should be together as we had been on all our other New Year's. We did manage to see some fireworks going off over Newcastle at midnight and shortly after that Rosalynde returned home. I always miss her when she leaves but on this particular occasion I felt very lonely as I watched her leave the ward; she turned as always, blew me a kiss and was gone. I rolled on to my back to ease the other pain and tried to cheer myself up.

At this point I should describe the conditions on the ward I was in and particularly the "climatic" conditions there.

It had everything yet in a way it had nothing because the end result was that patients were not comfortable and it was mainly a temperature problem. The ward was elegant, plenty of natural light and spacious. What more could anyone require?

To begin with, the mattresses were covered in plastic, which, of course, does not breathe. The pillows including the duvets and the mattress were all protected for obvious reasons by this method too. The result, sadly, was the patient over heated, especially during the night, and of course profusely sweated. The temperature in the wards did nothing else but exacerbate this problem; under floor electric heating saw to that and the windows, which were not the best design in the world, had to be constantly opened to cool things down. The temperature according to the thermometer was usually just below the 80s. I know it's a room full of sick people at various stages of treatment and recovery and they should be kept warm but it is these people who matter when it comes to the crunch and the balance was just not there.

My first night was dreadful, I woke in a sweat, all of it where my body was in contact with pillows and sheets and this continued throughout most of my long stay. In the end I slept on the extra towels Rosalynde had brought in, anything to separate me from plastic. All the other patients had the same comments but there was nothing to be done really and so it will continue in the name of progress. I may be beginning to appear bitter at this stage; I probably am because things became drastically worse.

I really don't remember much about the 24 hours in the Dependency Unit and even though I was on a drip during that period I was not told or warned about dehydration. Back in the main ward I began to feel an urge to drink, my mouth was dry, so dry in fact my tongue seemed to stick to the roof of my mouth. Unfortunately, at this time I was also feeling decidedly off-colour, nausea seemed to be beginning to dominate everything else, even the pain. This resulted in my developing a revulsion for water, too, which added to a growing situation. All this happened very quickly and for no apparent reason at the time except that it all stemmed from body fluid loss starting with the draining of at least a couple of litres from the pleura, followed by sweating in ''greenhouse'' beds, followed by the operation, followed by nausea and sickness and natural urination. I was dehydrating and no one spotted it in time except Rosalynde who complained to the sister on my behalf several times. I don't blame the nurses they always seemed understaffed and rushed off their feet although you would have thought one of them would have noticed my predicament or listened to Rosalynde's complaints. I blame someone higher than that who should have known better. If that someone ever reads this I just want you to know the extreme misery you caused me, the worry to my wife, family and friends and the delay it caused me in having future treatment, which was important to my continued survival.

I intend to complain to the Freeman Hospital in writing not because it can do any good for me now but it might help some other patient in the future.

Professor Proctor had called in to see me telling me they were still holding a bed for me in Ward 8 and he noticed my obvious decline. I think he may have had a quiet, tactful word behind the scenes because as soon as he left I was put on a drip and told to keep drinking. Not so easy to do at this stage, it had been allowed to go too far. When the medical staff discovered my predicament things started to move and fast. A doctor even rang Rosalynde during the night to explain that I had gone into renal failure, my kidneys had shut off to protect themselves and they had sent for a kidney specialist to come in and see me but they would ring Rosalynde again if she was needed. They then tested my urine and found the nitrogen content was rocketing up, in other words too much protein, my kidneys were not working properly; in fact they were failing. The "cure" was to stop eating food containing protein and drink large quantities of fluid and hope the kidneys would kick back into operation. That was easier said than done because of the dreadful nausea I was experiencing. I felt so low one night, lower than I've ever felt before that I remember whispering to Rosalynde as she leant over me to ask how I was, 'I feel so awful I wish I hadn't come through the operation. I wish you could just press a button and "switch off the light and end it all".

Throughout all this, although I didn't find out until later, Rosalynde played a strong hand behind the scenes, she was very angry at all my unnecessary suffering. She had confrontations with the Ward Sister and the young doctor, who on call for more than one ward that millennium weekend, insisting in the end on seeing Mr Forty, the surgeon in charge of my case. Finally things started moving but, in my own opinion, almost too late.

Even humour, however, can creep in at a stage like this. An amusing example happened a couple of days later when a couple of close friends, Peter and Patsy Jemison who were not aware that I was only having family visiting, came in to see me. Peter is a budding author but still trying to get his first book published. I asked him how his latest endeavour was going and he enthusiastically began describing his plot.

He had just finished and asked me what I thought about it when the food trolleys arrived and the smell wafted over to me. I knew immediately what was going to happen and grabbed with Rosalynde's help a sick tray from my bedside table then proceeded to vomit enthusiastically into it.

I looked up at everyone, very embarrassed. Peter, who has a dry sense of humour, said without batting an eyelid, ''Well, I've had some comments about my writing before but never anything quite so direct or to the point!'' We all burst out laughing, even me, who was feeling far from cheerful.

The sequence of events from that evening increased in pace and I hope I can remember everything clearly.

Everyone seemed very concerned and a strict monitoring of my fluid intake and output was kept. I was also given injections in connection with the kidneys but I do not know what they were. My legs and stomach began to swell as my body retained fluid rather than losing it in the natural way. I was beginning to look grotesque. I then had a visit from a Professor from the Renal Department, who was very pleasant and gave me the the following facts:

My creatinine level had shot up and had to come down in the next couple of days. Creatinine is a waste product normally cleared without any problem by the kidneys. In my case it was not being cleared and there was now some doubt as to whether the intravenous saline solutions and my own attempts to drink more fluid, were working. If things didn't happen quickly I would have to go on to a kidney dialysis machine, which was bad news and meant more needles and discomfort.

The turning point came almost on the point of arranging for dialysis and I was so relieved. At last something was happening in my favour. I had been warned that once the kidneys had turned the corner, I would be ''peeing'' profusely for a few days and in order to keep the momentum going I had to drink long and often to replace what was coming out. By then and even with the fluid retention I had lost a great deal of weight. I had arrived at the Freeman weighing 11 stone 3 lbs and was to leave it down to 9 stone 7lbs. I looked like a starving prisoner of war.

To make matters worse again the doctors decided I had to have a colestomy bag fitted to assist the urination and monitoring of the amounts. Although this was not as uncomfortable an ''operation'' as I expected I found it, personally, very embarrassing.

During this period, which was already traumatic, another and bigger bombshell landed and blew up in my face.

One Lump or Two

First, the surgeon who had operated on me came to see me. He told me that he was very pleased with the results and had cleared all the pockets of infection, it was just a question of the wound healing. The lung hadn't been damaged and had reflated successfully but unfortunately ………….. at this point I instinctively knew there was bad news to follow the good news!

An interlude from Hospital - lookuing at our old photographs

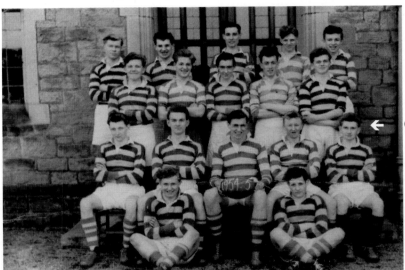

George

As a teenager playing for the 1st XV - Queen Elizabeth Grammar School , Hexham 1954 - 1955

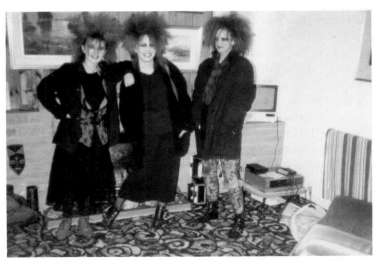

No, not MacBeth's "Three Witches" but an adolescent daughter (on the left) with her two friends going out to a "gig" in Newcastle, 1985.

136

Chapter 31
Worse News

The surgeon looked at me carefully before speaking further as though he was reluctant to go on and then he explained that he had found a small nodule in the lung and had removed a section from it for biopsy. The biopsy showed it was lymphoma. He was quick to say it was low grade, which softened the blow but only slightly. I don't know how many times I've been stunned by news like this but I've never become used to it. I have learned to control my feelings, however, and outwardly I didn't flinch. Inwardly it was very different. The disappointment flowed in. I had built myself up to cope with salmonella, which was bad enough, especially with everything else which had gone wrong but this really was a "bolt out of the blue". The surgeon's voice drifted back to me and I concentrated hard trying to listen to his next words. He had informed Steve Proctor at the RVI and presumably he would be in touch with me. He had also arranged for me to have a scan from the neck down to the groin and that would be sometime during the next two days.

The scan was arranged very quickly and as I went through that process, I couldn't help thinking what else would be unveiled. I felt reasonably confident that it would only be the node in the lung but I've learned from bitter experience never to count my chickens before they are hatched. When it was over it was back to the ward and the waiting game, often the worst part.

A couple of evenings later while Rosalynde was visiting me, Steve Proctor arrived and after the usual friendly greeting proceeded to draw the curtains around my bed which puzzled me somewhat. He then sat on the edge of my bed and broke the news. The scan showed that there were also lymph nodes in the spleen and liver.

I could tell Steve was upset at having to break this news to me. He had of course done this on more than one occasion but this time and like me he had thought all the previous symptoms had been related to the salmonella poisoning. Even though this had turned very nasty in itself, it still wasn't cancer and had given us all the false impression that things on that side were still under control.

He told me that had there just been the node in the chest, which was low grade, he could have treated it with Cyclophosphamide which had relatively few side effects. The other two nodes added a different dimension and there was uncertainty that others could be lurking elsewhere. Without further surgery there was no way he could tell whether the nodes in the liver and spleen were low grade and he felt treatment should be started as soon as possible. This unfortunately was hampered at that moment in time by the kidney failure, my severe loss of weight and the serious nausea I was still experiencing.

All this sounded very ominous to me and I said "This is really serious again isn't it?"

"Yes it is but I have been going over your files and comparing it with our records of patients we have been treating over the years on our database and I found something interesting and encouraging. One of my other patients has a history of reoccurrences similar to you – a series of low grade returns followed by a much more serious one of medium to high grade, which as you know I have to hit you hard with much stronger and more aggressive treatment. I treated this patient with a new drug in 1992, it was successful and on top of that he hasn't had any recurrence since.

There is, of course, no guarantee that this would produce the same results with you; everybody is different, but the drug itself is a powerful lymphoma cancer cell killer and it attacks low grade and medium to high grade cells wherever they are in the body and with a high rate of success".

I looked at Rosalynde, who smiled rather wanly at me, and then back to Steve and said "Thank you for being honest with me. It is a hell of a shock and it hasn't all registered yet". I tried to smile and make a joke of it by adding "do I pay my golf fees this year?" It was a rather weak joke but even hearing Steve saying, "of course you pay your golf fees", was a small but significant boost to my morale. What would I have thought if he had said "No!".

Steve then continued.

"The important thing is to get your kidney function back to normal, put some weight back on, improve your appetite and get you back to the RVI where we can start things rolling".

There were a number of things I felt I ought to be asking but I suppose I was still in shock at the news and couldn't think of anything. At times like this I also feel like being on my own, away from everyone so that I could collect my thoughts and work out how I was going to approach this new crisis in my life.

This is something Rosalynde and I have discussed before – my reluctance to share things especially unpleasant episodes. I am not really a talkative person, I avoid long conversations (except a good argument), I dislike the telephone, enjoy periods of being on my own, which is why I like going to our cottage so much and walking in the Cheviots. Strangely enough I write long letters – I seem to communicate better through the written rather than the spoken word. Rosalynde has often commented to various people on how much she enjoys reading my letters and said she wished I talked as much as the way I wrote.

The postmistress, now retired, from the village where we live, read my first book and commented to me that, while reading it, she felt that it was written as though I was beside her talking to her and she felt that all the way through. Other people have made the same comment since and maybe that was the reason for its popularity.

After Steve left Rosalynde took my hand in hers and said "I knew about the situation before I came today; Steve rang me at home and told me more or less what he's just told you. I just want you to know that I still have the same strong feeling that you'll get over this, that there's some purpose to everything that is happening to you. But, you, have to believe that too and continue fighting as you've done all these years".

Easier said than done even though what she said added another ray of hope in an otherwise dismal moment.

Later when Rosalynde left for home I sank into a real state of depression. "Not like you, George Walker" I could imagine people saying, "not the man, who has inspired so many people in recent years to fight back against all the odds. This is unworthy of you!"

My answer to that is simply "How much can one person take – it seems a never-ending series of vicious blows below the belt?" I must confess I no longer felt I was "Mr Invincible", in fact, I felt it was teetering on the edge of a long drop into a dark, threatening abyss and if I fell there was no way back.

This feeling stayed with me during the rest of my stay at the Freeman and I tried not to show it. I joined in conversation with fellow patients and my visitors and even taught a couple of them how to play cribbage, a game Rosalynde and I had learned in America and enjoyed playing very much. However, everything was overshadowed by what I had to face in the not too distant future.

I forgot to mention earlier that Steve had told me I would lose my hair again but other side effects would be minimal. This would be the third time and I was not looking forward to being bald again. The drugs would be intravenously fed into a vein and I would need a Hickman line implanted in my chest. I'd had one fitted when I had the autologous bone marrow transplant and it wasn't a problem and the real bonus was no more painful needles for extracting blood samples. I had needle injections every day at the Freeman Hospital, sometimes twice or thrice in one day and my arms and hands were sore and very bruised from the attempts – the Hickman line would save all that.

A Hickman line is a thin flexible tube which is fitted into a vein usually in the lower neck area. It has a self sealing end piece which enables needles to be inserted and a connecting tube for chemotherapy drugs, blood transfusions etc. It has to be kept scrupulously clean and flushed at least one a week to make sure it remains free of possible infection and working. It is a simple but pain and labour saving device. Dr Hickman deserves a pat on the back for this medical invention which has to be fitted by minor surgery – I am assuming it was a doctor who perfected the idea.

But all this was still ahead of me and I spent my last few days in the Freeman preparing myself for the ordeals to come.

I did, in fact, eventually find time to write a long letter of complaint to the Chief Executive of the Freeman Hospital outlining everything, which had happened, in much the same way as described in this book.

Unbelievably, I did not receive a reply or an acknowledgement and, after a

One Lump or Two

wait of 2-3 weeks, I wrote again sending a copy of the first in case the excuse came back that the first had not been received (both were by recorded delivery).

I received a prompt reply this time but the letter was written in such a way that it made Rosalynde and I very angry. It was what is normally described as a "whitewash". The only really useful point being made was that the surgeon had held staff meetings about my predicament, the emphasis being that every effort would be made to ensure that a similar situation would not happen again.

There was no mention of anyone accepting any responsibility for what had happened nor was there any apology from this very senior man for the distress and suffering his hospital caused me.

I wrote a letter in this vein back to him and would have thought more highly of the man if he had had the decency to reply (and promptly) with a simple apology.

I suppose this was too much to expect. Anyway, I hope lessons were learned and no-one else has to go through what I experienced.

I must emphasise that the surgeon and his surgical team did their jobs well and indeed I am very grateful to him for having the experience to spot the lymph node in my lung and do the necessary follow-up work before handing things over to Professor Proctor. It was the after-operation care, which was the problem.

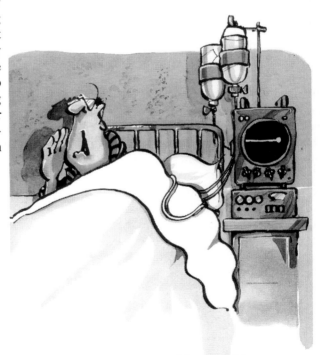

"Excuse me. The machine is making
a funny noise and the little light
is going in a straight line."

Chapter 32
Transfer to the RVI and a Slow Recovery

It was Friday, 15th January when I returned by ambulance to Ward 8 at the RVI. It was about 4.30 pm, daylight was just turning into dusk and, as it was my first trip out since before New Year's Eve, I was more observant than usual about the grey mediocrity of Newcastle's once mid-wealthy suburbs. There was a tidiness about the place though and after the bustle of Christmas, the roads and streets looked pleasantly quiet.

"Wait until tomorrow", I thought, "Newcastle at home to Southampton!"

The friendly faces of the staff at Ward 8 were there to welcome me back with the usual greetings "Thought you'd got away from us had you?" etc. I then settled in. I would have preferred to have gone home but needs be when the devil is about and this was a very safe sanctuary.

Rosalynde arrived later staggering as usual with goodies, drinks and spare clothes. But she was a welcome sight, as always, and although looking tired, proceeded to brighten things up. John and Eileen Thompson arrived later and we spent the evening chatting and laughing about old times.

I slept better that night than I had done for a while. It is not easy to sleep in ward 25 at the Freeman which is a very busy ward, half are heart patients, the rest are lung and there is a lot of pain around (and coughing) but the system works well and a steady stream move back out into the world to resume normal lives. Ward 8 was much quieter and although I woke early I didn't feel quite as depressed as I had been and, after a hot shower, I met the day staff accompanied by Lorna Renwick, the Ward Sister and we swapped stories.

As these things happen, the night staff nurse was giving out the patient history and I found myself staring at her surname, which was Fiddes, on the lapel badge she was wearing and it triggered off another of those amusing incidents from my past, which I'm always looking for to brighten up the story of fighting cancer.

I thought they could do with a laugh, to cheer them up to face a long day, so I interrupted the medical dialogue with something more light-hearted and told them this story:-

In my probationary year as a school teacher part of the process was to be observed at work by the Headmaster. Mine was a "stickler" in the old fashioned sense and not one with a great sense of humour.

A colleague of mine, who was also in his probation year, was teaching English to his class and had formed the class into groups and was taking group reading when in walked the Head, unannounced. There is always an immediate reaction to probationary teachers when this happens, the mouth goes dry, you become nervous and your brain starts racing "Have I got my notes?", "Is everything in

One Lump or Two

order?", "What do I do now?", "Don't panic" and so on.

The Head pulled up a chair beside him and joined his group. "Carry on were his supposedly calming words "Just imagine I'm not here".

The young teacher looked around the group in a panic and his eyes landed on a young lad called Fiddes. "Right, Stiddes!" he blurted out "You fart!" It is easy to imagine the shocked silence described to me, which was followed by an outburst of laughter and, apparently, even the auster Head joined in.

Whatever else happened though, reading lessons in his class for the rest of that year wouldn't be quite the same. The nurses found it very amusing and Staff Nurse Fiddes, I imagine, would never quite see her name in the same light again.

After that amusing incident, I was destined to stay in Ward 8 for almost a fortnight as the staff helped me to recover from the trauma of the Freeman Hospital.

Rosalynde and me at school camp (the summer holidays 1962) South West Scotland

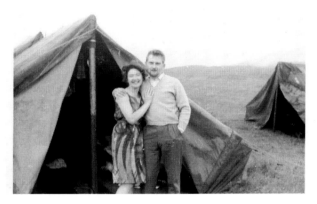

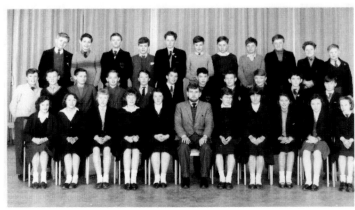

My favourite class (Prudhoe High School 1962)

142

Chapter 33
Ward 8

Ward 8 is where all the patients requiring treatment for blood-related cancers and other blood illnesses are treated. It ranges from bone marrow transplants to doses of chemotherapy and various other treatments followed up with essential after care. Once discharged, follow up and check ups, blood counts, blood and platelet transfusions are often carried out at the Haematology Centre, which is now based on Ward 6a. Steve Proctor has succeeded in bringing once fragmented departments into 3 wards on the same floor, a great improvement for everyone.

Ward 8 is run by Sister Lorna Renwick, one of the most dedicated and caring sisters I have ever come across. She is Scottish, but I won't hold that against her, and comes from Jedburgh in the Borders – my favourite area (both sides – English and Scottish).

Her work and example are reflected in all the staff under her charge; they are all very aware that they are fortunate to be under her guidance and training. She is a tireless worker, often going home well after her statutory time. Nothing is a bother to her and she never dishes out a job I haven't seen her do herself, even to mundane, sometimes menial tasks.

Throughout all this her sparkling humour shines through and she always has a cheerful encouraging word for everyone regardless of the situation. She is known to have a bite, or is it a bark, and when this occurs on rare occasions, the staff are soon aware of it and they do their best to appease the wrath that is to come.

Lorna reminds me of myself and the way I've seen teachers changing over the years. In my early days we never counted the extra hours we did after the school day ended and weekends away with the youngsters were taken as a natural extension of the job and unpaid. Standards appeared higher then too – teachers don't seem to dress smartly any more, especially male teachers and this is strongly depicted in the television plays about schools; no ties, sweatshirts, even jeans and so on. Standards between teachers and pupils have changed for the worst too and, of course, disciplining a child now is like "walking on eggshells".

My first teaching appointment was with a Headmaster of the old school – fairness, discipline, high standards in all things were his creed and we all responded to it, staff and pupils.

Lorna is of the old school in exactly the same way. Some nurses now seem to be more career orientated, degrees and qualifications being the driving urge rather than the real vocation of caring for the sick. It is not their fault – it's the way society has changed – they are under tremendous pressure in their work and they deserve the perks of promotion when it comes along, I was no exception to that myself. I don't mean any of this to be derogatory, I have a great respect for nurses and the marvellous work they do, the very long shifts they work and the care they put into it. It would, however, be to everyone's advantage if the best of these changes were taking place for the good of the people in their charge – the patients and I'm sure most nurses

Ward 8 nurses and ancillary staff have this attitude and I'm sure it is all down to Lorna's influence, which hopefully means when they move on to other wards or hospitals, those traits will go with them and may even influence things for the better when they do.

Lorna has one drawback as far as I am concerned – she hates having her photograph taken. There isn't a single photograph of her in my first book – I failed miserably to capture her for posterity. I'll keep trying this time however, and maybe she'll appear in this book.

I cannot end this chapter without mentioning the doctors, the old hands have already been mentioned but in these last few weeks I've seen a new generation of young doctors doing their training as House Officers on Ward 8 and if they are anything to go by the future of health care is in good hands, at least with them.Between them, the whole team worked on me to build up my strength and stamina in preparation for the chemotherapy treatment to come.

Steve Proctor had told me the various drugs and treatment, which he had decided was the best way to tackle the situation and he has written it out for me in such a way that non-medical people like myself will understand it. His account is as follows:-

The treatment of non-Hodgkin's lymphoma for a given patient must be individualized. There are some thirty different varieties of disease which present in different organs and there is the possibility of evolution from one form to another.

George's disease presented with a large abdominal mass in 1988. At this stage it was a mixture of intermediate and low grade. Treatment was with chemotherapy/radiotherapy and autotransplant.

Over the years recurrences were localized areas of "low grade" recurrence treated in a low key manner with radiotherapy. When in the last 90s a recurrence showed characteristics of "high grade" tumour under the microscope further aggressive chemotherapy called CHOP for short (four drugs) was used and radiotherapy.

Subsequently the new drug anti-CD20 (Rituximab) was used when in trial phase to damp down any residual "low grade" tumour. After this came the unexpected salmonella infection, which in the event, was to mask a further lymphoma recurrence.

On recurrence after the chest operation in 2000 the situation was difficult with disease in the liver and spleen being the brunt of the problem. The use of the "Newcastle cocktail" (IVE – Ifosphamide, VP16 and Epirubicin) was required. This combination was first used by us in lymphoma in 1991 and since has become established in the UK as a treatment with much potential in the management of non-Hodgkin's lymphoma.

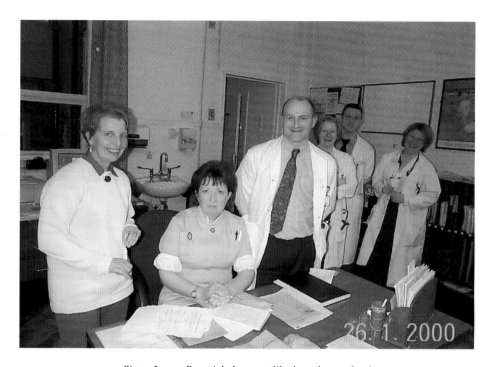

Sister Lorna Renwick does not like her photo taken!

Chapter 34
Dominic

During those days in Ward 8 I fluctuated between bouts of depression and moments when I seemed to mentally rally but these were few and far between. Times, which helped, were when I made contact with other patients on the ward. Several of them passed in and out within a day or two but there were others, like myself, who were in for an extended stay. What disturbed me was noticing the age of most of them – young in comparison to myself. There was John, a bus driver, who was suffering from leukaemia but fortunately for him he had a brother whose bone marrow matched his own and he was in preparation for a life-saving transplant operation. A long road lay ahead of him but with every chance of survival.

There was also Chris, who was in his late twenties and from Alnwick. He was in the next bed to me and was going through some debilitating chemotherapy treatment and showing all the signs I knew only too well; the worse being vomiting from a stomach which no longer contained anything to bring up and thus causing great discomfort. I tried to cheer him up but he was going through a really bad time and escaped when he could into uneasy, but long periods of sleep. I became friendly with his wife, Susan, who sat by his bed reading while he slept.

Amazingly, it turned out that she had just recently recovered from the same illness as her husband, lymphoma, and was now in the best of health. Two people not related, except by marriage, with the same life threatening illness – one of life's cruel coincidences except that they were both

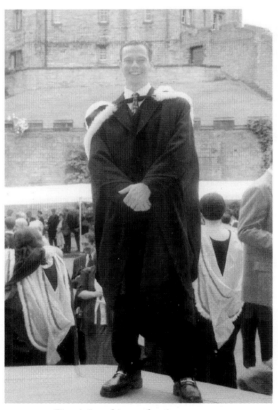

Dominic at his graduation ceremony

146

able to benefit from each other's experiences. He like John was also lucky in that his brother was a matching donor and once the disease was under control he would reap the rewards.

The good news that followed was both John and Chris went through all their treatment which was successful and they are back to living normal (well, as normal as can be expected) lives. When I met the couple from Alnwick at our 11th Last Night of the Proms later that year both Susan and Chris were both looking very healthy and very happy.

It is not always like that though and another young man I met during my hospital stay was going through a similar but not so successful episode in his life. His name was Dominic, he was in his early twenties and bursting with life and enthusiasm. He was so cheerful and easy to approach that I struck up an immediate bond with him, at least when the opportunity arose. His bed always seemed surrounded by his family and friends and it was usually only early mornings or late evenings when we had a chance to chat together.

I have already mentioned I was very low in spirit, still desperately trying to recover from earlier health problems at the Freeman and facing the miserable, fear-filled weeks that lay ahead. Rosalynde, God knows what I would do without her, was battling away in her own calm, unflappable way, keeping me going with her smile and unquenchable faith in our future together. Dominic somehow added to that and gave me that extra boost that I needed and how important that was did not really emerge until he told me how serious his situation was.

It took me all the way back to July 1988 when I was told I only had approximately 12 weeks to live. Dominic was going through a similar traumatic experience made much worse by his age and that he had everything in life going for him. He had just gained a good honours degree, a new job in Newcastle working with disadvantaged young people, which he obviously loved and he had just bought his first house. Then the unexpected happened. He became ill and was diagnosed with acute myeloid leukaemia that was not responding to treatment as had been hoped.

If I had not become friendly with him I would not have realized how desperate things were. He was always smiling and unbelievably cheerful, everyone was drawn to him by his strong outgoing personality. I hope I was able to help him a little in the way he helped me and which he would probably never realize. I felt I did because when he realized how serious my situation had been and with very little hope left, there I was still alive. Rosalynde brought me a copy of my book, which I loaned to him and I think this helped him and his family too.

He became very interested in our concerts and the fundraising we did for cancer research. His mother, Rosalind (another Rosalynde – not quite the same spelling but certainly with the same compassion and drive) was also very interested and although the family lived at Penrith in Cumbria, she said she would love to organize a party to come to the Last Night in October. I said we'd arrange tickets etc. for her and I would expect Dominic to be there too.

During my long recovery back at home I called in to see Dominic when I attended Steve Proctor's clinic for check-ups. He was always as cheerful as ever though we talked about his situation and his fears. He told me that the new treatment he had been having had seemed to work for a while but the illness returned with different symptoms. He was hoping he was going to be given some other treatment and he had lost his hair again and looked thinner. My heart went out to him and it didn't really help to know that I was responding to treatment while he was struggling.

Later in the summer when I was almost back to normal we travelled to Cornwall to see Ben, Suzanne and Anthony and then on returning home left three days later for the Isle of Arran. No sooner had we returned from there then we headed for Norfolk. We were making up for lost time and the good weather and exercise (golf and cycling) worked wonders for me. My hair slowly grew back and I at last began to feel normal.

It was almost September when we settled back into a routine in Newcastle and we soon became heavily involved in preparation for our 11th Last Night of the Proms, scheduled for 21st October. Everything was hectic but going to plan when we received a telephone call from Rosalind Niedt, Dominic's mother, who broke the sad news to us that Dominic had died.

It was an awful shock because I always felt that Dominic had the strength and will to pull through but sadly it was not to be.

I wrote to his mother shortly after the phone call telling her what he had come to mean to me in the short time I had known him and I hoped that she and his father, his sister and student friends would still come to join us at the concert. I felt it would help them tremendously to experience the wonderful atmosphere, which was generated there, and I'm sure it would help them in their grief. Rosalind replied they all intended to come and they would see us there. I also asked her permission to mention Dominic in my end of concert speech as a tribute to him, which she agreed to without hesitation.

Dominic, you are out there somewhere in the "space" we all wonder about. I don't know whether you are aware of the impact you made during the short but very fruitful time you were with us on this earth, I like to think you do.

Rest in peace knowing this and that everyone you came into contact with loved you for what you were – a truly remarkable and very brave young man.

Chapter 35
Returning Home

The day finally came when I was told I could go home; what would follow after that would be the long period of treatment, spread over at least two to three months as described by Professor Proctor.

Steve had decided that as the salmonella poisoning and kidney scare had weakened me, the first treatment would be in two stages rather than one. Instead of three drugs, I would have one and a half days treatment and follow that up with another one and a half days when he saw how I reacted to the first. Before that I had to build up my strength and body weight. This was helped by a course of anabolic steroids – the substance banned for athletes and body builders, which is a muscle builder and appetite improver.

After looking in the mirror when I stripped off the first evening home, I could see clearly why I needed it. I looked awful, absolutely skeletal and what flesh I had was loose and wrinkly just like a very old man. I couldn't help feeling revulsion at what I'd become. The change in a few weeks was frightening. I had to make every effort to return to my normal, fit and reasonably athletic-looking body – athletic for a 62 year old man that is!

That night Rosalynde and I moved close to each other in bed. The first time we'd been together properly for weeks. We put our arms around each other and just held on. I breathed in the clean, slightly scented smell her hair always has and felt her body warmth creep over me. It was good to be back but even that was spoiled, but only slightly, as I became conscious of the warm, firm flesh of her body pressing against my skin and bones. I couldn't help thinking "God, what must she think she is holding" and I felt embarrassed at the thought. But Rosalynde is Rosalynde and she gave no indication, whatsoever, that I was anything different from the young, normal man she had married. I could feel she was glad I was back; her love came through as strongly as it has always done and I soon relaxed and enjoyed the comforting feeling until we eventually fell asleep.

I woke early – hospital routine is hard to break – and was lying on my back suddenly overcome with an awful feeling of despair and depression as everything bad, which had occurred and was going to occur, flooded into my mind. I stared at the ceiling willing these thoughts to go away, desperately trying to think of something positive and cheerful to help me but I couldn't. Rosalynde must have also been awake because she put her arm over me and said "What's wrong George?". How she knew I don't know because I was just lying there, everything unpleasant was going on in my mind, not hers or so I thought, but that is one of her gifts – a remarkable sensitivity especially for people needing help.

One Lump or Two

It was too much for me, everything just welled up inside me but I managed to blurt out "Rosalynde, I'm frightened, I don't know how I'm going to find the strength to get through the next few weeks. I just don't think I'm going to come through them. Everyone thinks I'm a sort of superman, that no matter what happens to me I can bounce back. I'm not, I'm just an ordinary bloke trying to stay alive". At that point I felt my voice going and the tears starting. I turned my head away so Rosalynde wouldn't see the state I was in but the tears turned into sobs as I struggled in vain to control myself. Rosalynde pulled my head round to face her and stroked my cheeks, wiping away the tears.

"George, regardless of what you think or feel, people do respect and admire you for the way you have fought your illness. You have inspired many people to do the same and you should be proud of that. We both know the next few weeks aren't going to be easy but we've got each other, we have Marc and Roxanne, wonderful friends and neighbours, all very much behind you. People have been praying for you and think about you all over the country. Look at all the cards, letters and phone calls we've received. You can't let them down – we're going to win".

I wasn't convinced but I felt much better and a little more under control.

"I still think everyone expects too much from me and they forget this has been going on over 13 years now. How much longer can I keep it up? I'm dreading the next few weeks, the treatment and having to face everyone for the third time without any hair and the way I look. It makes me stand out like a sore thumb. Unless you've gone through it no-one knows the mental trauma you have to cope with and you know the number of times it has happened to me".

"Yes I do but you've come this far and done so much good on the way. You have to keep going, you know I'm always there with you".

I did know that only too well. It's easy being swamped by my own fears and problems to forget the burden Rosalynde has had to carry throughout all of this. The weeks of travelling back and forward to the hospital, the ups and downs and swings in my moods as I crawled my way through the maze of mental anguish and physical deterioration. Coping with the many, many enquiries which flooded in, usually by telephone and usually in the evenings when she needed a well earned rest.

I've said before that my illness has become a very public illness because of our charity and the involvement with the North East Proms and other concerts. Subsequently, when things go wrong our many followers and supporters are naturally interested in my progress. If people weren't I'm sure we'd be very hurt and we really do appreciate the concern and love which is expressed every time things go wrong. It's Rosalynde who acts as the buffer and copes with all the enquiries in her friendly, sociable way. I do hope these comments do not put people off keeping in touch in the future – their good wishes have meant a great deal to us. It really boils down to me and my strongest wish that life for us could turn back to the normal way it used to be but that is wishful thinking and if that is the case, so be it.

I don't often cry, although I have been moved to crying in a number of ways over the years. A sad moment in a film, even a happy moment can affect me, certain music moves me. I remember when Janice Cairns made her first appearance for us and sang "O My Beloved Father". Her father was sitting right behind me and I know she was singing it to him. I was moved to tears then. These tears were for other people. I don't cry for myself but I did this time and I was glad Rosalynde was there when it happened. We talked on for quite a while afterwards and became very close. I wish I could be like that more often, very close I mean, but I always seem to be in a hurry, engrossed in a hundred other things and too busy to think about something which is really more important. I will try harder – impatience and thoughtlessness should be listed as the 8th and 9th deadliest sins.

Probably the first sign that I was finding a spark of my former energy and determination to be in control of myself again occurred later that day when we had a serious talk about the 5th Suzanne Manuell Concert which was looming up over the horizon – the 8th April to be precise. We had already assumed that we might have to cancel it because of all the unexpected circumstances. As many of the preparations had already been seen to before I went into hospital, it seemed a pity to call it off. I really had no idea what state I'd be in during the next few weeks and if I had any sense I should have dropped it. In the end I suggested to Rosalynde that we leave it to our concert-goers to make the decision for us. We had a pile of stamped, addressed envelopes sent to us after the Millennium Concert in November. All we had to do was send the printed leaflets along with an appeal letter explaining the position and stating the concert would be either on or cancelled depending on everyone's replies. Rosalynde did the appeal letter and signed it. We made enough copies of it with the help of our neighbours, John, Ina and Rachel Wagget, and we sent them all off in the post with a decision deadline for the middle of March.

The response from our supporters was overwhelming and we went ahead with the concert plans even though it was a struggle and I had no idea what sort of condition I would be in when it took place.

Chapter 36
The Treatment and "Fun" with a Wig

Steve Proctor has already mentioned the "cocktail" of three drugs I was due to have as soon as he felt I was up to it and that, in fact, was only a few days after my return home. The break itself, though, had been a great help to me, giving me the opportunity to release the pent up feelings and emotions, which had built up inside me since Christmas. More importantly I was able to release them in the privacy of my home and with Rosalynde.

I still had to steel myself to enter Ward 8 even though the greetings were as warm and friendly as they have always been. Rosalynde was with me as usual and once I was given my bed space, we unpacked my things and she stayed on for a couple of hours to help me settle in. We had our usual games of cribbage, a game we learned in America and have become quite addicted to ever since.

I was given the drugs on the next day. They were fed intravenously and took several hours. I didn't feel any immediate side effects but felt sleepy during and afterwards. I stayed on for another couple of days for blood tests and observation and was given the usual tablets to help the body deal with the toxicity of the drugs.

Finally they let me go home but I had to report each day to the haematology clinic for blood tests and I was given boxes of tablets to take home to continue with the "rescue" treatment. The tablet regime was quite complicated especially remembering the different times they had to be taken and whether before meals or after meals or with food or without food and so on.

There was a three week gap between each treatment and it was during the second spell that my hair began to fall out. I have described several times how traumatic it is to lose one's hair from chemotherapy so I won't describe it again. I was, however, not looking forward to it and discussed it several times with Rosalynde. I had also watched some of the women in the ward who wore wigs when they lost their hair and they looked very realistic and obviously helped them cope with it better than us weaker men.

I then had the idea that perhaps a wig might help me and spoke to Steve Proctor about it when we had a moment together. Even that was embarrassing but having mentioned it I felt I had to give it a try. Steve was very helpful and understanding and suggested I talk to Sister Renwick, who could arrange for me to visit a wig shop in Newcastle to try some out if I felt like going ahead with it. Everything would be confidential and very discreet or so he said.

I did talk to Sister Renwick and she gave me the address of the shop she dealt with and also a voucher enabling me to have a wig paid for by the National Health Service – an unexpected bonus. I decided to go ahead with the idea and would make an appointment on my return home after the second treatment was completed. On that particular day Steve led his staff of doctors on the ward round, most of them young and some I had come to know quite well.

They gathered around my bed and after the usual comments about my treatment and blood test results Steve said in a rather loud voice "Did you speak to Sister Renwick about being fitted for a wig?"

I felt so embarrassed; I thought everyone's eyes upon me and very probably no-one was even interested but I didn't know that or think that. I just wanted to creep away. Pure pride, of course, but so much for confidentiality and discretion!

I mumbled something in reply, looking up at him from the bed at the same time. I didn't feel like looking around the group and was very relieved when they moved away.

It all appears an amusing story now but at the time it was a very sensitive area for me for all the reasons I have mentioned earlier and, once again, I must emphasise that this was the third time I was about to lose all my body hair and I absolutely hated it!

I did actually go ahead with acquiring a wig but I rarely used it. It did, however, come in useful when I was away from home where people didn't know me. I would wear it then and it actually gave me quite a psychological lift even though I never really felt 100% comfortable with it. I could never rid myself of the thought that everybody I met would immediately think "Oh, he's wearing a wig!" Not a terribly important concern really but it does show how easily things like this can affect people.

I did learn something about wigs though. The lady at the shop couldn't have been nicer. She understood my predicament and proceeded to describe the ins and outs of wig wearing. Apparently, it definitely is easier for women and it is more acceptable for them. Most women have good thick hair which doesn't usually thin with age. They also change their hairstyles quite frequently according to fashion. The quality of wigs has also improved greatly over the years. So, when a woman wears a wig it is not so noticeable and, in fact, is often not recognized at all as a wig.

This is not the case for men. It is not possible to make a wig to look like hair is thinning or spars as the membranes of the wig show through. Consequently, unless the man has already had a crop of thick, luxurious hair, which is rarer the older he becomes, when he suddenly appears with an eye-catching mop of hair, it is immediately noticed by everyone who knows him.

The wigs I looked at and tried were all like this and even though I found two which were exactly my colouring, they were so good I almost looked like a young man again. There was finally one in particular which Rosalynde and I thought was the nearest I would find to my normal hair and the wig lady even managed to thin it down a little with some deft scissor work – this was after I had decided to have it, of course.

One Lump or Two

On the occasions that I did wear it I found it helpful but more often than not I reverted to the tried and tested "baseball" type hats that most other men wore and just stuck it out again. It was an experience though and I hope that this account will help any other male person who finds himself in a similar predicament and is as touchy as I am about losing his hair. There was one small consolation , it gave me an idea that would help me face the audience at the forthcoming Suzanne Manuell concert but more of that later.

Between the second and third treatments I had a CT scan and waited with fingers crossed for the results. They were good and things started looking up for the first time. I even thought treatment number three might not be necessary and that would be a real bonus but the answer was an emphatic no. I had to complete the full course just to make sure but I felt the weight easing off my

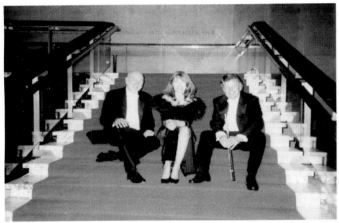

Above:Suzanne & Anthony with special guest, David Haslam
Below: Suzanne & David performing

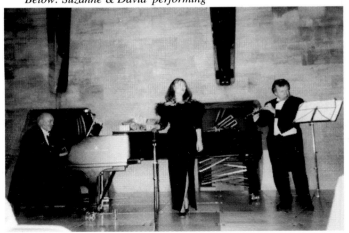

154

shoulders for the first time and life took on a different meaning.

Suzanne's concert was just before my final treatment and the preparations for that, hectic though they were, acted as a relief from everything connected with the medical world. I still had my daily visits to the hospital for blood tests but the scan results made them much easier to bear.

The concert was excellent with another full house. Looking back now I'm glad we didn't cancel it even though I had to face everyone without hair and beard for the second time with that particular series of concerts.

The idea I had from the wig episode went down well in my welcoming address. I borrowed a large curly, jet black, Afro-Asian wig from one of Roxanne's friends and her psychedelic sunglasses. I already had one of those dreadful Scottish ginger wigs with a beret stuck to it. I then told the audience that one of Steve Proctor's sidelines was selling tastefully designed wigs to his patients under discreet and strictly confidential conditions – wigs which would not cause embarrassment and attract unwanted attention.

Steve, of course, was sitting right in front of me with his wife, Sue, wondering what was coming next. I then placed the hideous Scottish wig on my bald head which drew a spontaneous burst of laughter from the audience. An even louder burst erupted when I swapped it for the gorgeous but outlandish Afro-Asian wig telling everyone that you received a free pair of sunglasses with that one and proceeded to wear the dazzling psychedelic glasses.

I don't know whether Steve saw the connection with the wig incident in the hospital. I doubt it but it was all good fun and it broke the ice for me thus helping me through the rest of the evening.

Suzanne's guest that evening was David Haslam, principal flautist and conductor with the Northern Sinfonia. I wasn't sure how the flute would go down with this type of concert. Before that the instrumental guests we had were both violinists which I think is probably the most popular solo instrument there is. I now think the flute must be a very close second as David played beautifully and his choices of music were just right for our audience and they loved them.

No sooner had our guests departed, all the bills paid and the euphoria of a wonderful evening's entertainment had died down then I was back in the reality of life and steeling myself for the final treatment. Eventually I even had that behind me and distressingly thin, no hair, an even more damaged immune system but hopefully cancer free, I gathered myself together and set out on the long road to recovery.

Chapter 37
Recovery and Making Up For Lost Time and Another Concert

Recovery was slow, not surprisingly after what I'd been through but the early summer weather helped and we spent some time at our cottage, tidying the garden and, of course, some tentative games of golf at the Hirsel Golf Course at Coldstream. Actually, the garden didn't need much work because Emily, Linda and Ruby, our cottage neighbours who knew about my predicament, had joined together to help us out during our long absence. This is what we have come to expect from friends like that and we were very grateful. The cottage itself had survived the winter remarkably well – no roof leaks and no dampness as we had kept the night storage heaters on low over the winter and it was a pleasure to stay there again. Some of the seniors at the golf club did not recognize me when we saw them on the course because of the hair loss but were pleased to see me alive and golfing when they did – they knew what I'd been going through.

Back home there was more work to be done especially in the garden but I had help from John, a gardener friend who did a few hours for me when he could and we made steady progress in that direction. There was also the mid-summer concert arrangements to be done – advanced booking forms sent out along with publicity as we always started selling tickets for the "Last Night of the Proms" in early July. This was mainly because of the long school summer break, when many people disappear on holiday with their families, which is a dead period for selling tickets. We like to start early so by September we know where we stand and still have time to sell remaining tickets – a strategy which has always seemed to work.

Someone commented to me when they realized what we were involved in that no-one would think we had just spent the last few months struggling against a life-threatening illness. It was as though it had never happened. Not quite true but that's how it appeared to other people. I think they often wondered what drove us on when we should simply have just spent the rest of our retirement enjoying ourselves and avoiding the stress and frustration of running a registered charity. I can't answer that – I just don't know really except that I've seen so many people die from cancer or suffer from it that I just cannot turn away. I know Rosalynde feels the same way too but I sometimes feel guilty at dragging her into all this but knowing her as I do, I don't think she would have had it any other way. We've both aged during the last few years and I sometimes feel terribly responsible for all of it.

We do, however, have our moments when we can escape from it all and that is exactly what we did as soon as we had set the advanced booking process into action.

With a ¼ inch of hair and beard beginning to appear we first headed to Cornwall again to see the "Cornish Mafia" and we had a great time with them, first at Ben's home before he flew off to America to join his friend, Suzie Crofut. Then on to Suzanne and William's farm where we stayed for the rest of the time and had our return game of golf with Anthony and William – Cornwall versus the North East – and we beat them again even though Anthony showed none of his usual generosity with Rosalynde by giving her six feet puts, every shot had to be played!

Our next "escape" was to Arran fairly soon after we had returned North. Ian and Jean MacMillan, who had loaned us their lovely croft on the North West coast of Scotland, also had a large caravan on the Isle of Arran.

Ian rang to say he was there on his own as Jean had to go and visit a sick aunt on the mainland. Why didn't we drop everything and come and join him. He gave us travelling details, the address of the caravan park and within a couple of days we were there and had a fabulous time. The first week was with Ian, then he left to join Jean allowing us to stay for a further week and the weather was glorious every single day. We explored the island by car and walking. Every morning we swam in the park's pool. I struggled at first because of the chest operation but gradually increased the number of lengths each day and began feeling my lungs improving with the exercise. We played most of the golf courses on Arran and our golf improved too. In the evenings we sat on the caravan decking eating and drinking in the balmy air and watched the herring gulls diving for fish as the sun slowly sank in the azure blue sky – heaven on earth.

It was hard to leave that lovely island but we had to step back into the world again but it was with fresh heart and a spring in our steps. The horrors of the first part of the year started to fade into the distance. On top of that the ¼ inch hair growth was longer and thicker and my beard was looking pretty good too which gave me an added boost.

Our third escape was to revisit Norfolk and join our friends, John and Catherine Baugh, in their caravan. Naturally the golf gear went with us but we also took our cycles – Rosalynde loves cycling in Norfolk, I wonder why? Could it be because it is very flat? We stayed in the Sandringham area first and we paid our first visit to the Queen Mother's residence there. What made it even more interesting for me was seeing the houses, the church and the beautiful grounds where Captain Frank Beck and his Sandringham Company, comprised of men who worked on the estate, lived and worked before they were shipped to the Dardanelles where all but one man was killed by the Turks.

Only months earlier we had seen the TV production of "All the King's Men" which depicted Captain Frank Beck, played by David Jason and his men and the mystery which surrounded their disappearance as they marched into battle. Legend said they were covered by a cloud and when it lifted they had disappeared. The reality of it was they were captured and shot. It was a very moving and finely produced programme and to be standing in front of the memorial of these men at Sandringham itself so soon afterwards made it more real to me than just a television drama.

Before returning North we spent another few days in the southerly part of Norfolk revisiting some of the places we had been too a few years earlier.

It was a great summer for us, something we both desperately needed and if and when the friends we shared those holidays with read this, it gives me another chance to tell them how much we enjoyed their kindness, their company and the pleasure of being with them in those beautiful places.

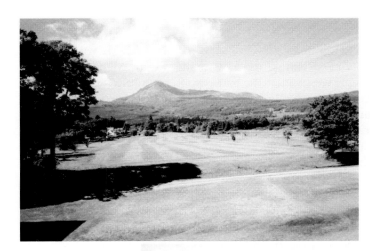

Brodick Golf Course on Arran looking towards Goat Fell

The caravan where we stayed on Arran

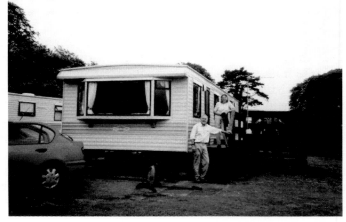

Chapter 38
The First "Geordie Prom" of the New Millennium

During those early months of 2000 when things looked so black for me, a large question mark hung over the future of our concerts and, therefore, our charity. As I have explained earlier, we managed to save Suzanne's concert because it was so imminent but many people, on hearing about my struggle to survive again, thought the "Last Night" would not take place and that would probably mean the end of it. It is very difficult to resurrect something after a two year gap no matter how successful it has been.

Fortunately, it wasn't the case and my earlier chapter about Dominic Niedt, the courageous young man I met and came to know so well in Ward 8, and the effect he had on me, made Rosalynde and myself even more determined than ever to continue with our fundraising efforts to beat cancer.

I must admit though that, after those three wonderful holidays, it was very difficult to pick up the reins again. If we hadn't set the ball rolling with the publicity and booking forms being distributed in June, I'm sure the temptation would have been there to have said, "let it go, people will understand". But that is all hypothetical, we didn't and the response to the advanced booking forms was so fantastic we were soon in the midst of all the preparations as though nothing had happened to threaten it.

There were two other bonuses for us also. First, our charity's accountant and auditor, Peter Willey, a great supporter of our concerts along with his wife, Pat, had recently moved his offices into our village and he offered us a spare room at a very modest rent. We are still in the process of using it to the full because so many things appertaining to the charity are more convenient from home and 12 years of habit die hard. However, it will become a great bonus to us eventually and we are slowly emptying our house of all the accrued files and paperwork, which almost took over our home.

The other was an offer of help from David and Jennifer Cranston, which we gladly accepted, and they were a godsend during the weeks leading up to the 12th Last Night Concert and, indeed, still are.

David, now retired, was Chief Executive of Northumbrian Water piloting it through the traumas of privatization. He supported Ian MacMillan's bid to bring the company into our sponsorship "team" after we met on a skiing holiday and the company has supported us ever since. The Cranstons have become very good friends of ours, as have Ian and Jean. David's experience and his meticulous attention to detail, recording and forward planning have added a new dimension to the "Walker" system. Their detailed knowledge of opera and classical music has also been a great help – they are both opera and concert

159

"buffs" regularly visiting London and other prestigious centres of music in their leisure time.

I efficiently keep files on everything connected to the charity and the concerts but the planning and build up to every concert is stored in my mind and tends to leap out as I move through the year. That is okay if I'm fit and well and around but if not then Rosalynde and whoever else might be involved, would find themselves all at sea because of the intricacies of it all and my personal connection and relationship with the key people. Not good practice for the reasons already stated but it is now all logged with instructions, fine detail and in chronological order so that in my absence, for whatever reason, someone can pick up the strings.

Things do change each year, however, and things can go awry but it is there to follow and manipulate to advantage.

On top of becoming good friends, David and Jennifer, like us, are keen bridge players and we have started weekly matches at alternative houses. The score is 6-6 at the moment so we are holding our own.

The 11th Last Night of the Proms on 21st October 2000 was another sell out. The programme and performance was excellent. The wonderful fanfare "Sprach Zarathustra" by Richard Strauss (Space Odyssey 2001) opened the proceedings of the first half, which ended with the fabulous 4th movement of Beethoven's 9th Choral Symphony involving all the singers and choirs.

The lively, foot-tapping orchestral piece "Hoedown" from Aaron Copeland's ballet "Rodeo" set the tone for the more jolly, "party" atmosphere of the second half and this was where Rosalynde and I persuaded our conductors and soloists to make some daring changes to the programme. We moved into modern times, completely out of tradition but the gamble paid off and the audience loved it.

The gamble was to perform songs from the end of the 20th Centrury even moving gently into the pop and musical scene. Queen's brilliant "Bohemian Rhapsody" specially scored for orchestra and choir by Len Young was the first big step. An artist friend created a full size figure of Freddie Mercury,

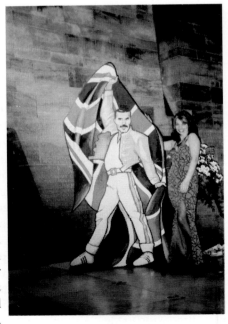

"Freddie Mercury" in performance at the Proms 2000 with Suzanne

posturing in a gorgeous sparkling "outfit" as only he could and waving a Union Jack over his head. This stood at the side of the stage covered in a black cloth until the right moment when he was carried out, allowing me to unveil it after saying a few appropriate words. He stood beside the conductor throughout his most famous piece and the audience gave "him" a rousing reception obviously enjoying the showmanship of it all.

Also included were songs from South Pacific and Carousel sung by Sir Thomas Allen and Suzanne Manuell. Then the more recent hit songs of Andrew Lloyd Webber from Evita and Phantom of the Opera etc sung by Janice Cairns and Blake Fischer, a handsome, young tenor from Australia, who was making his debut for us.

Blake was studying opera at the Royal Northern College and was introduced to us by Rachel Luxon, Ben Luxon's young and very talented, opera singing daughter, who was also studying at the college. We were originally going to have a "Sir Thomas Allen and the Three Sopranos" programme (we had that idea before Pavarotti's concert which was on TV at Christmas that year) but Rachel couldn't make it. She had just secured an important three month contract with the Welsh Touring company so we had to re-think the whole thing.

Blake was a great success. He had a very lyrical tenor voice, perfect for musicals and his operatic arias etc in the first half showed his full versatility. He made the most of this love duet with Janice and their kiss at the end brought howls of delight from the audience.

More appreciation of his talent was to follow when he sang a verse in both Rule Britannia and the Blaydon Races. I had bought him a traditional Australian hat with the dangling corks, which he kept hidden till then and when it appeared there were more howls of appreciation. His "piece de resistance", however, was, unknown to anyone else, his own "Aussie" version of his verse in Blaydon Races. He was adopted as a new member of the team from that instance and I'm delighted that he is going to sing again in the 12th proms later this year.

Another great moment for us that evening was the arrival of Ben Luxon, the man who started it all with us in 1989. Everyone knows the tragedy of the last few years, when he became profoundly deaf bringing an illustrious international singing career to an end. He has, however, never missed one of our concerts and has never missed appearing on stage where he always receives a tremendous ovation. There was a huge question mark over this one and I even paid a tribute to him in the souvenir programme just in case. He made it to everyone's delight, joined us in the audience for the first half and the singers for the second when he sang splendidly in "Rule Britannia" and "Blaydon Races". His record remained intact and I'm working on yet another appearance for him this year. In the finale I decided to sing my speech and asked Ben and Rosalynde to join me. Without Ben it would have been impossible, as I cannot sing in tune. We sang the first song as a trio which was based on the song "Anything they can do we can do better" referring to Sir Andrew Davies's sung speech at the real "Last Night of the Proms" earlier in September at the Royal Albert Hall and Steve Proctor, who sang his speech at the beginning of the evening. Ben and I sang my second as a tribute to Rosalynde.

"She's a grand lass and a bonny lass and she likes hor beer, they caal hor Rosie Walker and we're glad that she's heaor" etc, etc. The audience loved it and reacted with a tremendous burst of applause and laughter.

What a great miss this wonderful concert would have been if it had been cancelled as it so nearly was.

The "bucket collection" afterwards of loose change donated as people left the theatre and subsequent postal donations from those who somehow didn't see them in the crush, reached just over £3,000, more than double from any of the previous 10 concerts; a tribute from everyone there for a marvellous evening's entertainment by superb performers and all for cancer research and patient care!

Rosalynde, who always has the last word on the stage, said and very appropriately, "The Geordie Last Night of the Proms has become one huge, happy family, having a great night out together and all for a great cause – what could be better?"

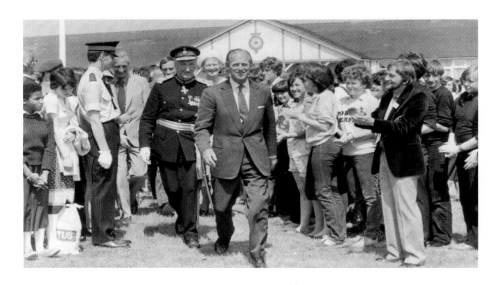

Looking back again - me welcoming the Duke of Edinburgh to the 25th Anniversary celebration of his Award Scheme at Harrogate Showground (1981)

Chapter 39
A Mild Stroke?

I was going to bring this story to its close after the 11th Last Night of the Proms concert but strange events have taken place since then putting me into the RVI for an enforced stay of seven days. It was, however, a neurological ward this time not Steve Proctor's ward, although he had a hand in placing me there. It was a confused and very frightening time and even now I am having great difficulty in piecing it together. Fortunately, Rosalynde recorded most of it in her diary, which she has meticulously kept up to date for years now; in fact, I don't think I could have written either book without referring to her record of events.

Many people were aware that I was trying to write a sequel to my first book and I was coming under more and more pressure to get on with it. Once all the euphoria of the success of our October concert had died down I decided to make a big attempt to get on with it. I decided the best place was at our cottage on my own with no disturbances from the outside world (except for two games of golf which I managed to squeeze in).

So on the 15th November I set off with paper, biros, diaries and food to my Cheviot refuge. The only happening to break into this regime was a quick return to Newcastle on the Saturday to attend Rachel Wagget's 30th birthday party with my family. Rachel's family are neighbours and very close friends of ours and Rachel and Roxanne, our daughter, grew up together and have remained firm friends too. Rosalynde thinks the first signs of my strange behaviour started when I returned home for the party but as I have always been spontaneous and unpredictable she thought nothing of it. The party was a huge success, packed with young people enjoying themselves and what was even more enjoyable was the way they accepted us "oldies" into their world of deafening music and carefree bonhomie.

Next day found me back at the cottage frantically trying to force myself into writing again. The quietness of the cottage seemed even quieter after the explosion of fun the night before and the writing did not flow as easily as usual.

Monday found me back on form but Tuesday slowly turned into a nightmare and with no real warning. I had risen early, laid and lit the fire, had breakfast on a tray as the table was covered in papers where I had been writing.

After washing the breakfast dishes, I sat at the table and picked up the story from where I had left off the night before. After writing a few lines I stopped and stared at the last few words, which ended in the middle of a sentence. I could not find the words to end it. I re-read the previous sentences but still couldn't think of the words to go on. I left the table and wandered around the room, not unduly disturbed but thinking a stretch of the legs and slight distraction might help. It didn't, in fact, it was worse and this time I found I was having difficulty in reading and understanding any of it. The thread had snapped and I couldn't bring it together again. I had heard of writer's block and wondered if that was what I was experiencing.

But I sensed something was wrong; something I appeared to have no control over. I made one last effort to bring things back to normality by going outside and started finding jobs to do in the bracing air from the Cheviot Hills. This needed no real concentration; after over 30 years spent in these parts, I know from sheer practice the jobs that needed doing. I chopped sticks for the fire, piled fresh logs at the door, swept up the autumn leaves, raked the gravel drive, filled the wire cages with nuts and seeds for the birds and eventually washed and polished the new Almiera Tino, I had recently purchased, until it shone.

Feeling refreshed and invigorated, I had sandwiches and a cup of tea and rather nervously returned to my writing – to no avail, I could not read what I had written. I decided then to leave off writing and prepare for returning home instead. I was due to return early on the Wednesday morning anyway to keep an appointment with Steve Proctor and after lunch with Rosalynde, I was returning to the cottage to carry on with my writing. Rosalynde was going to join me for the weekend.

I decided to keep to these arrangements. I cleaned and tidied the cottage, packed my things and retired to bed for an early night, thinking I probably only needed a good night's sleep. The bedside alarm woke me at 7 am and after laying the fire and a quick breakfast I set off for home with my few things. I left all my writing on the table, food in the fridge assuming I was still returning the same day.

All seemed well until I felt an overwhelming urge to close my eyes and sleep. Realising how dangerous this was I pulled into the first layby that appeared, switched off the engine, settled back in the seat and promptly fell asleep. This happened three more times until I reached home at Westerhope and this worried me as I do not normally feel sleepy when driving unless it is a very long journey.

Rosalynde was more or less ready to join me for my visit to the RVI but we had time for a drink of tea and a chat before we left. I started to tell her about the writing "glich" and seemed to be perfectly lucid in doing so but Rosalynde said she couldn't understand what I was saying. At this point I found I could hardly hear what she was saying, which became worse as we tried to keep the conversation going.

Eventually we both realized something was definitely wrong and decided to leave it until we could talk to Steve Proctor. Fortunately or unfortunately, depending on how one looks at it, I was still confused and hard of hearing by the time I saw Steve at his clinic. I tried to explain my predicament to him but judging by his expression I wasn't making much sense and I could barely make out his replies. Rosalynde then took over and did most of the talking. After a very thorough examination consisting of movements of my fingers and arms, which I had never done before, Steve told us that he thought I'd had a mini stroke and he felt I needed to have an urgent brain scan if it could be arranged. He made a couple of phone calls and said "We're in luck they can squeeze you into a vacant slot at 2.30 pm, they've just had a cancellation. I suggest you go home, have some lunch and come back for the scan".

"On no account", he added "is George to drive until we've completed all the tests".

He was really talking to Rosalynde as I could barely hear what he was saying.

At 2.30 pm we were back at the RVI and heading for the CT scan room, another place I had visited often during the past 12 years. The staff there recognized me and, after a few friendly words, I lay on the "bed" of the scanner and was moved slowly into position. This time only my head and shoulders disappeared into the machine and I found myself listening to the pre-recorded instructions as my head was moved a fraction at a time to enable the machine to take a "slice" at a time as it produced an image of my skull and brain to enable the radiologist to see and diagnose any abnormalities. It was quick and painless and we returned home after being told the results would be passed to Steve Proctor within a few days and he would probably contact us.

It was Marc's birthday next, "What a build up to it!" I remember thinking. Marc wasn't coming home from Edinburgh until the weekend though we had sent him a birthday card without mentioning anything about my problem. The next few days passed by without any further deterioration but I was still unable to write anything or read anything for that matter. Whenever I started reading the words would just disappear.

We took Marc out for a meal on the Saturday evening, his partner Catherine had remained in Edinburgh as she had an urgent piece of commissioned work to complete. We explained to Marc and Roxanne about my predicament but as I didn't do anything untoward I don't think they realized how serious it was becoming.

We saw Marc off on the train to Edinburgh on the Sunday morning then drove to the cottage, stopping at the Black Bull Inn at Bowsden for a delicious Sunday lunch on the way. It was only a quick trip to the cottage to collect the food I had left there, switch off the fridge, check everything else and then straight back home. We had decided writing and the cottage were out until things had improved.

On Monday morning Rosalynde and I went to the Westerhope Golf Club for a round of golf. I didn't play too well and found that I couldn't see the ball on long shots, consequently I lost about three that morning, which was unusual for me. I also found I was having difficulty with my balance when swinging the club and in choosing the right club to use. In fact, it became difficult to distinguish which club was which. The only consolation was that it was a lovely day and we both enjoyed the exercise.

That evening Ben rang from America where he was visiting Suzie Crofut and other friends. He was landing at Glasgow airport on Wednesday where he would collect his car and stay with us for a few days en route to Cornwall. Steve Proctor also rang that evening to tell us he'd made an appointment for me with a colleague of his, Dr David Bates, a neurological consultant and asked us to meet him at the clinic on the Tuesday morning and he would take us to meet Dr Bates. I wondered why he hadn't mentioned if he had received the CT scan results and assumed he hadn't as yet. Unfortunately, it wasn't as easy as that because a little doubt crept into my mind exactly as it does on similar occasions. "Was the news about the scan so serious he didn't want to talk about it on the phone and if the results were good then why didn't he tell me and put my mind at rest?"

This had happened to me several times and no doubt to many other people but we just have to "sweat it out" and wait for the news which is much easier said than done!

Next morning we met Steve as arranged and, before we met Dr Bates, he told us the CT scan showed no signs of tumour, which had been his main concern. I sighed inwardly with relief as that had been my main concern too but I had not mentioned it to anyone, not even Rosalynde.

"I cannot comment on any signs of brain damage if you have had a mild stroke that will be for Dr Bates to comment and we're going to see him now", said Steve before leading us from his office to Dr Bates' office further down the main corridor. To be honest I am assuming it was down the main corridor as I don't think I could find Dr Bates office even now when things are back to normal. I just followed Steve and Rosalynde with a "woolly" confused head, unable to make out what they were talking about and on top of that the sides of the corridor seemed to be disappearing.

Chapter 40
Deaf, Blind and Scared

We liked Dr Bates as soon as we met him. After Steve's introductions, he shook both our hands with a warm smile, which made us immediately relax. Steve left and Dr Bates started his examination, which began with my rather confused attempt to explain what had happened to me. Rosalynde filled in most of the gaps when she saw me struggling to find words.

"I could find no signs of brain damage on your CT scan, which rules out a stroke of any kind", he explained. "Would you mind if I brought my registrar to join us?"

We had no objection and Dr Bates left his office returning in a few minutes with his colleague, who I was to see more of over the next few days. She and Dr Bates then asked me many pertinent questions and put me through physical tests similar to those given by Steve but with others added.

During all this I tried my best to sound intelligent and alert but I felt all the time that I wasn't saying things in the right way or order. I would start to say something then found I couldn't finish it and then I would try again but it would sound worse. Rosalynde, of course, completed the picture for me and at the end Dr Bates said he would like me to come into his ward for a few days for further tests and observation. He had no beds available at that moment but would be in touch as soon as he could offer one.

We left it at that and then after seeing Steve again to report our progress, we left for home to wait for the next move.

Next morning our neighbour, John Wagget, came over to ask me if I'd like to join him for a walk. John, a former paediatric consultant at the RVI and now retired like me, wasn't aware of any of my difficulties or so I thought but a few minutes later I discovered that Rosalynde had mentioned it to him and his wife, Ina, and they were concerned.

John took his car and this was when things started to accelerate and made me realize that there was every possibility that I was going deaf and even worse blind! John had decided to drive down to Newburn where the bridge crosses the River Tyne to the south side between Blaydon and Ryton. On the way there I was looking at the scenery and suddenly realized I could not recognize anything. This was along a stretch of road, which I knew as well as anywhere else around the Tyne where I had lived for nearly 40 years. I didn't mention anything to John but sat quietly trying to control the panic, which was threatening to overwhelm me. We finally stopped at a car parking area on the bank of the Tyne and I dismounted from the car, looked around and said to John, "Are we anywhere near the river?" John confirmed that we were. It was right in front

167

of us. I could see John and on looking down I could see the tarmac of the stopping place and the path but I couldn't see anything else. I then explained to John what was happening to me and he said that Rosalynde had mentioned it previously to him.

After that I walked alongside John following the river path in a westerly direction towards Wylam. As we walked I could only see things that were very close to me but beyond that nothing. I never saw the river or the surrounding countryside throughout the walk. I remember seeing some houses as we passed close to them and it was near there when we turned off on to another path to return to the car. Before that we arrived at a pub, which I saw as we drew near to it and John took me inside to the bar commenting that the pub had its own micro-brewery adjacent to it.

I lost some of my tension, which had been building up on the walk and recognized a man at the bar, who had served with me during National Service, a very long time ago. I introduced him to John as "Ollie", his nickname really which was derived from his surname, Holliday. After a couple of beers, John Wagget seemed to grow restless and suggested it was time to leave. What I didn't know was that while I was talking over old times with Ollie, John had slipped out of the bar to the telephone and had rang Rosalynde. He told her he could not persuade me to leave the pub and he had an urgent appointment to keep with Ina. Rosalynde said she would come down in our car and help.

John then returned to the bar and, at that stage, I realized John wanted to leave and after saying goodbye to "Ollie" I followed John outside to his car.

On the way home John apparently met Rosalynde coming in the opposite direction and flashed his lights. Rosalynde turned round and followed John home. I was completely unaware of this as I was back to the reality of John's car and was concentrating on the bewildering, unrecognizable scenery which was passing by the car window.

That evening Ben arrived and joined the team of people who were very worried about me and my stranger than usual behaviour.

I have forgotten to mention that Dr Robinson, from our local general practice, called to see me at home following word from the hospital. He examined me and he too was baffled by my condition but was happy with the way things were being speedily put into action at the RVI. He told me to make an appointment at the clinic for a cholesterol check which I did and at this point I was awaiting results.

The day after the river incident was uneventful until about 4 o'clock. Ben had driven over to the Freeman Hospital to see a Dr Miekle, who had been trying to help Ben with his hearing problems. Ben was needing advice on further treatment he had been having, which involved another large dose of steroids. It seemed that steroid treatment was about the only medication which could keep total deafness at bay but the downside to this was the side effects from long and sustained doses of the drug.

Meanwhile Rosalynde was preparing a meal for the evening and I cannot remember what I was doing. I do remember her saying she needed more potatoes and, without telling her, I slipped out of the house to buy some. I don't know why but I think I wanted to prove I was still capable of some initiative of my own.

It was growing dark by this time but I seemed to find the shop easily enough but once inside I could not work out where the potatoes were and I had been in that shop many times. Rather than ask the assistant, I left the shop, crossed over the road, where fortunately I could see the Pelican crossing, and entered the larger supermarket named Aldi. This was against all my principles because we had fought long and hard to prevent this supermarket being built there when there were already three supermarkets close by. It was a village eyesore and I had vowed never to shop there. As I was determined not to go home empty handed I broke my vow and entered the store. It was almost empty and there seemed to be only one person on till duty. I walked down the aisles confidently thinking I would see the vegetable display area but I couldn't find it nor could I recognize any of the other display areas. I gave up, walked out and returned home to meet a worried and angry Rosalynde. She had just returned from the Waggets after looking for me everywhere; except, of course, the new supermarket, which she knew I would never enter! I think John and Ina gave us some potatoes and poured some oil on troubled waters.

Ben returned with the news that he had to continue with his steroids for the time being so he too was a little "down in the dumps" like the rest of us.

There were three things happening during the next two days which we were looking forward to and they had all the ingredients to cheer us up. On Thursday evening we had been invited to a 19th and early 20th Century Paintings Exhibition in Newcastle and we were going on from there to the City Hall. This time we had been invited by Andrew Bennett, the new Chief Executive of Northern Sinfonia. It was an evening of Bach music and what made it special for me was that Bradley Creswick was performing and David Haslam was conducting. Both musicians had become a very important part of our "Proms" team and both had been our guest artists at Suzanne Manuel concerts.

The art exhibition was a disaster for me. When we arrived I was fine but, by the time I mounted the stairs to the exhibition rooms, I could make out the paintings on the walls but the details were blank. Absolutely strange, frustrating and even worse, terrifying. I could make out people around me and hear conversations but could not understand any of them. Ben and Rosalynde had wandered off on their own so, without letting on, I just followed the flow of the other guests. I finally found Ben and Rosalynde; they were together and bargaining with the dealer for a painting of a horse by Isaac Richardson, a member of a famous North East family of artists. Ben asked my advice about it, which I would normally have gladly given but I had to admit to them that I couldn't really see it. The short of the matter is that Ben bought it after agreeing a discounted price and we left for the City Hall. On the way there my sight and hearing seemed to return, to our relief, and I entered the Hall on a much happier note. We were seated about eight or nine rows from the stage in the middle; a good position for vision and hearing. I really enjoyed the first half but by the end of it I felt things beginning to change.

This spread into the interval when a number of friends came over to greet us. I tried to be sociable but felt extremely awkward. Several weeks later, when we met some of these friends again, they remarked how vague I had appeared to be and, of course, they presumed something was amiss.

There certainly was, during the second half I could not see the stage or the orchestra, nor could I hear what they were playing and they were only a few yards (or metres depending on how old you are!) away.

On the way home, with Ben driving, I persuaded them to call at the Jingling Gate, a local pub, which had just been refurbished. I fancied a pint and was curious about the alterations. It was also an attempt on my part to cheer everyone up. Everything seemed to be normal. I thought I had regained my sight and sound after leaving the City Hall. At the bar I ordered drinks and scanned the area to see the alterations but I couldn't make them out. I seemed to be in a little world of my own with only Ben and Rosalynde with me. I turned and was able to see the barman, who had completed my order. I paid him and tried to pass the drinks to them but I could not distinguish them on the counter and had to ask Ben. After that I could only feel for my pint in order to have a drink.

The whole baffling thing about all this is that I wasn't blind in the normal sense of the word and neither was I truly deaf. I imagine blindness to be black, with no emission of light or signals to the brain. That wasn't the case with me. I was aware of light and I could make out objects but at the height of things I just simply wasn't aware of them. I also learned from experience that it seemed to occur when I had to concentrate on things e.g. the meetings with the doctors, the art exhibition, the concert, the walk with John Wagget and so on. Between these spells and others like them I was relatively normal.

When I woke up in the morning things were normal but within half an hour or so the cycle began again and usually when having breakfast, again concentrating on something. This is probably too wide an assumption but there was a pattern there to see, if you'll pardon the pun! I was also still falling asleep during the day especially when watching the television. This did not affect my night-time sleep as it sometimes did when I had the odd nap during the day.

Anyway, next day, Friday, Ben set off for the long drive home to Cornwall diverting to Buxton, to hear his daughter, Rachel, sing at a concert there. The phone rang just as he was leaving. It was the RVI and a message from Dr Bates stating he had a bed for me and wanted me in that afternoon. After Ben left, we packed a few things and headed for the hospital yet again.

We reported to Ward 11, the neurological ward, where I was shown to a single room, to my pleasant surprise. I was expecting an open ward and was wondering how I would be able to communicate with other patients if and when I lost my sight and hearing, which was a frequent occurrence now. It was a pleasant room and the staff were very friendly, rather like Ward 8, where I had stayed on more than one occasion.

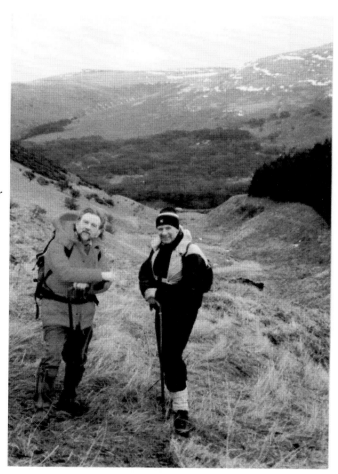

Introducing Steve Proctor to walking in the Cheviots

Chapter 41
A Light in the Tunnel

Rosalynde helped me to unpack my things and this is probably the only time I hadn't brought a book or writing paper with me simply because there was no point.

Rosalynde left rather quickly and I found out later that she had been asked not to stay too long and also to keep visiting and visitors down to a minimum. Apart from tests, they also wanted me to have a complete rest.

I was left to myself most of the day except for staff dropping in for information and delivering meals. The ward doctor came to see me and I went over everything I could remember while he made notes. During that interview I felt my vision and hearing go and told him so. At that point he left as, I assume, I wasn't making much sense by then.

I did not sleep very well that night. All my previous hospital stays kept flashing through my mind, particularly the unpleasant ones and I began thinking what would happen to me if I did not improve or, even worse, I lost my sight and hearing completely. It was a sobering thought; a lonely world of my own, no more golf, no walks in the Cheviots and visiting our cottage would never be the same. I would never hear music again, the concerts would collapse and this second book, which I was beginning to enjoy putting together, would never be finished. I felt very lonely that night and experienced similar moods as the rest of the days and nights went by. One small consolation was that this whole episode had pushed cancer way back down the queue and for the time being I had more important things to worry about.

The doctors had told Rosalynde I had to rest and rest I certainly did. The days were long and boring, the evenings and nights seemed even longer but gradually and with the help of half a sleeping tablet per night I settled in to the routine. During the next six days I rested mainly on the bed interrupted only by members of staff and the evening visit of my family. The tests I had were in depth and one, in particular, helped to ease my mind a little. This was a lumbar puncture, which I knew in advance I had to have. This consisted of a fine needle inserted into my spine to draw off a tiny quantity of spinal fluid. I wasn't looking forward to it after having so many needles piercing my body on many other occasions. Actually, it wasn't as bad as I expected. I had to turn on to my side and the doctor inserted the needle carefully as I steeled myself to take it. She must have felt my tension because she said "Relax it's all over". I was surprised as I expected worse to come. The doctor explained that the spinal fluid would show any signs of an infection or virus attacking the brain. Later in the week I was informed that it was clear – more encouraging news.

On Sunday Marc and Catherine, who were having a break at our cottage, came in with Rosalynde and Roxanne to visit. I could see and hear them when they arrived but I warned them that it might change. Sadly it did and slowly I became aware that they were disappearing and I could no longer hear them. It was a very depressing experience and similar occurrences during the rest of the week drained more confidence from me each time.

I learned how to return to my room after visiting the shower room and the toilet. If any readers have watched the interesting police series "Second Sight" on television, during January and February 2001, the Chief Inspector's dilemma with his failing eyesight and occasional flashbacks always reminded me of the experiences I am presently describing. He would use his hand along the corridor wall in the Police Headquarters to find his office. I could walk perfectly well to the toilet, which faced me at the end of the ward corridor but sometimes when I emerged I had to do the same action, hand along the wall and count the doors of the other rooms until I found my own room. I also learned to recognize the wallpaper pattern in my room and small notices, which read "WARNING VERY HOT WATER" etc. If I lost my sight I knew it had returned when I could read these notices.

Television was another good indication. If I started to watch it when feeling normal, the picture and sound would disappear within about five minutes reinforcing my earlier theory about concentration triggering the condition. I also discovered that if I lay on the bed and fell asleep when I woke up everything was back to normal. I started timing this and it averaged at about twenty-five minutes. I also realized I didn't have to sleep, just lie back, close my eyes and relax and try not to concentrate on anything. This action never failed and I told the doctors who noted the details.

Just before my second weekend in hospital Dr Bates told me he'd managed to book me in for a MRI scan at the Newcastle General Hospital on the following Monday and that would be the last of the tests. MRI means Magnetic Response Imaging and is a very sophisticated form of scanning parts of the body, especially the brain. It produces much greater detail, even of the fine tissue and is more effective than the usual CAT scan. I think there is only one of these in the North East and, therefore, long waiting lists but I had been given a cancellation.

I wasn't looking forward to another long weekend "confined" to a room so I asked if it would be possible to go home on the Thursday afternoon, organize my own travelling arrangements to the MRI scanner on the Monday and then wait to hear the results of the scan at home. The doctors agreed with me that the times between the "attacks" were widening and I promised to rest at home, which seemed to help them make up their minds. The decision rested with Dr Bates and, after consultation with him, I was told I could go home. I rang Rosalynde, who arrived by car within an hour and I was on my way home.

It was wonderful entering our home after eight frightening days in hospital and even more so when everything I looked at was clear to see and my hearing seemed back to normal. I had only one slight attack earlier that morning, which was disappointing in itself but it didn't last very long and, in my desire to return home, I hadn't mentioned it to anyone. I slept well that night and enjoyed wandering around the house and garden after breakfast. I felt so good I persuaded Rosalynde to join the ladies at the Golf Club for a few holes of "winter" golf assuring her I would come to no harm during her absence.

After Rosalynde left I began to feel restless. It was a very pleasant morning, I'd had no problems with sight or hearing that morning so I thought I'd go for a short walk around the village but decided against it as so much traffic pours through Westerhope these days. I felt like going into the country but Rosalynde had taken the car. Then I had an idea – why not a short bike ride out into the countryside around Westerhope where there are some very pleasant easy routes. The temptation was too strong to resist so I checked the bike and set off through the village. I headed for Kenton Bank Foot where there was a quiet route to Ponteland through the village of Woolsington and then back home – about nine miles.

All was well until I reached Kenton Bank Foot and suddenly as I approached the T junction to turn left to Woolsington, the inevitable happened and I cursed myself for being so irresponsible – my sight and hearing just "switched off!" It had taken me no more than about seven minutes to reach the outskirts of Westerhope but it took me well over an hour to find my way back home.

At first I just stood at the road junction, holding the bike with my mind racing in all directions, trying to decide what to do next. The good news was I knew exactly where I was but cycling home was out of the question as I would be on a very busy road all the way. There was no way I could contact Rosalynde, I was on my own!

I remember thinking "Come on you daft b......d, you've got yourself into this predicament, now get yourself out of it!"

And so, I did the only thing I could, I set off walking, pushing the bike at the same time. I had to cross the road first to make sure I was on the right side for home – only twenty or so feet but it seemed like a mile before feeling the curb with my feet. I kept waiting for the bang as a vehicle hit me, but I made it. After that it was a long, slow process of following the curbstone, touching it with the inside foot to keep me right. It was daunting every time I reached a road junction, I had to stop, wait, then go for it, trying to then find the curb again once across. The worst part was trying to decide when I reached the final turning into Highfield Road where we lived. It was on the busiest stretch of road through the village itself towards the Newcastle bypass and, unfortunately, on the opposite side of the road. Fortunately, the village Post Office is actually facing it and I could just recognize it, blurred though it was, when I finally reached that point. I stopped there wondering how on earth I was going to cross the road. I was beginning to hear slightly better by then and could make out the constant hum of traffic but the thought of stepping into it filled me with dread.

I then closed my eyes, leaned against the garden wall next to the Post Office, tried to relax and hoped I would regain some sight. Nothing happened for about 20 minutes and then I opened my eyes for about the fourth time and I could make out a permanently sited flower trough at the edge of the path and people passing close to me in both directions. A lady with a small child came into vision and I quickly blurted out "Excuse me but this may seem strange me standing here in cycling clothes and holding a bicycle but I have just lost my sight and I cannot cross the road".

The lady stopped and seemed concerned, not put off by the slight absurdity of the situation much to my relief. I quickly explained my predicament and she very kindly took me along the pedestrian crossing and helped me across the road and back to the road leading to my home. She wanted to see me all the way but I needed to do that part on my own and she understood. After thanking her, I walked up Highfield Road counting the houses until I turned into our drive and the safety of home. Rosalynde hadn't returned from golf and I debated whether I should tell her about my escapade knowing full well what her reaction would be but I thought it was important to tell her.She was furious, of course, and could not accept my strong desire to try and be normal again after everything I had been through but she softened as I explained that no harm had come to me.

It was quite a blow to the growing confidence that I had been experiencing and the hope that the whole strange incident was over. I also began worrying about what the MRI scan would show during the following week. Maybe it would show that something very serious was lurking in my brain – a sobering thought. So the worry was back and another long wait began.

What did in fact happen was exactly the opposite. From that hair-raising cycle ride till this moment of writing, about four months, I have never had another recurrence of either sight loss or hearing loss. The MRI scan was clear much to my relief and in the subsequent follow up session at the RVI both Professor Proctor and Dr Bates came to the same conclusion. The only explanation, which made sense after every test possible was clear, indicated that I was suffering from mental exhaustion and the brain was reacting in an unusual way.

In Steve's own words he said "The brain was SWITCHING OFF. If you couldn't see or hear then you couldn't do anything; nature's way of slowing you down perhaps but it's also a warning!"

He then proceeded to warn me that if I didn't slow down, reduce the charity work and try harder to cut out much of the stress, there was no guarantee it wouldn't happen again and, if it did, there was also no guarantee it would clear up again. Good advice but easier said than done, especially as I had been so moved by the death of the young man, Dominic, that I had committed myself to continue fundraising in front of 2500 people at the last concert. I had also committed myself, at the same time, to finish this story and have it published in time for the next Proms Concert in October 2001. I had dug and pit and jumped in again!

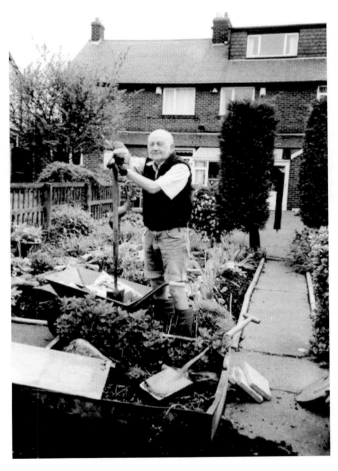

No hair but still gardening - starting the new garden design for our 40th Anniversary
Anniversary in August 2001

Chapter 42
An Amusing Incident with the Police

Somehow I must find space in this story to describe my brush with the police and how they thought I'd escaped from a hospital for the mentally ill – absolutely true! After the trauma of the last few chapters this will add some cheer and a few smiles.

Over the years, Rosalynde and I have explored many avenues in the field of complementary medicines and therapies and tried many of them. It was not in any way in competition with conventional medicine, which I have always acknowledged as playing the major role in my continued survival. We were more interested in anything that helped to boost the body's immune system, and general all round health to combat the debilitating and harmful side effects of chemotherapy and radiotherapy. Behind this, of course, was the hope that in doing so it might just help to stop the disease returning. Yoga, exercise, healthy eating, a balanced intake of vitamins, relaxation and meditation were some of these and probably the strangest of them all was Qi Gong; some people might describe it as the weirdest.

It is a special Chinese therapy and involves complicated body movements all designed to stimulate the body's energy field and help you to combat illness. Rosalynde and I attended a course and I concentrated, particularly on a special method of walking, which was developed to help people with cancer or who had survived cancer. If any reader saw the first television programme about me, "George and Geordie Proms", they might remember me talking about and demonstrating it in our garden. I had my leg pulled about it several times afterwards. I carried out this strange form of walking for three years for anything from one to two hours per day – outside in the fresh air and sunshine when possible. I even did it in Norway and France before skiing when it was freezing. Skiing time was too valuable to miss so I arose earlier than anyone else and did it before breakfast outside the hotel. I even did it around the swimming pool of the superb Dan Hotel in Tel Aviv, Israel. It was less embarrassing in France than Israel because the freezing, early morning conditions made sure I was the only idiot wandering around outside. The weather in Israel was different and even though I was at the pool, very early, I was soon being watched by early swimmers and with great curiosity. I saw and heard one Israeli tap his head and say to his gorgeous, bikini clad partner "He has to be a crazy Englishman!"

The walk is difficult to describe with words but I'll try to create a picture. It begins with facing the sun, brushing your hands from above your head down your body and breathing rhythmically and deeply as you do so. Then you begin to move forward swinging both arms from side to side as you set off. As you do this you breathe in quickly twice and then release the air slowly; this goes on every time you take a step. Your head turns to the right and left following the swinging of the arms. All in all, it is not a normal method of walking anywhere except on your own when you can then relax and enjoy it. When I could do it this way it was fine but there were times when I could not avoid people and I would wince inwardly whenever I approached anyone.

One summer's weekend Rosalynde and I were staying at her sister's home in Scotby, a village near Carlisle and, of course, I had to do my Qi Gong. According to the Chinese therapist, who taught me, it was essential to do it every day. On the Sunday morning after we arrived, I set my travel alarm and rose about 6.00 am deciding to make a very early start before any of the village folk were out and about so I would not be noticed. It was a beautiful morning so I dressed in tracksuit bottoms, t-shirt and trainers and crept quietly downstairs without disturbing anyone. Rosalynde was awake but said she would do her exercises in the garden at a more sensible time and snuggled down in bed.

I decided to have breakfast on my return and went to open the front door but couldn't find the key. I went to the back door but couldn't find that key either. So rather than wake Avril and George, her husband, I carefully climbed out of a window, pushing it to afterwards and set off. I hadn't intended Qi Gonging though the village and was going to walk to a farm lane which wended its way down to the River Eden. There and back was about four miles and very pleasant and probably completely deserted at this time of the morning. However, everywhere I looked the curtains were drawn and nobody was stirring so rather than waste half a mile I switched into the Qi Gong walk. The only time I had to stop was for a car at the A69 main road which joined the M6 just outside Scotby. It was only a solitary traveller and I was soon across and entering the lane to the River Eden.

As I "waddled" gracefully down the lane towards the first bend swinging my arms enthusiastically in time with my legs creating the strange mincing sort of step, which adds to embarrassment of being watched, I became conscious of a large police car (the jam sandwich type which we all recognize immediately) turn off the A69 into the Scotby road I had just left.

I remember thinking "I wonder where he's going so early on this lovely, peaceful Sunday morning", then promptly forgot about it.

About three or four minutes later I heard the sound of a car engine approaching from behind and swung over to the side of the lane to let it pass, assuming it was the farmer. Imagine my surprise when out of the corner of my eye, I saw the same police car slowly edge past me until the driver, whose window was down, drew level with me. It still hadn't dawned on me that I was the target because I just kept going, until the policeman said "Good morning, sir, are you alright?"

"Good morning", I replied, "Yes, I'm fine, thanks".

"What a friendly young man", I thought, still walking and swinging away. The penny still hadn't dropped and the policeman then said "Would you mind stopping for a moment, sir, so I can ask you a few questions?"

Thinking something must have happened in Scotby, which I might have witnessed, I stopped and turned to face him. I suddenly realized he was looking very uncomfortable and seemed unsure of what to say next so I smiled and waited.

"I'm sorry to have to stop you but we've received a complaint from someone in Scotby Village about a patient who has absconded from the Garlands Hospital, which is nearby and the description I have been given fits you, I'm afraid". I knew from George and Avril that this hospital was for people who were mentally ill and the whole thing suddenly became clear – penetratingly clear. I couldn't help it at that point and just burst out laughing, which startled the policeman, so I hastily tried to "clear my name".

"Sorry, I didn't mean to laugh but I think you will see why when I explain", I said trying to look as normal as possible. I then proceeded to tell him more or less what I've just described in the last couple of pages. By the end, he too was smiling and we continued to chat about the situation, which he found amusing too.

"The person, who rang, was apparently quite upset at seeing you wandering through the village waving your arms and looking from side to side and was convinced you were out of your mind; I can imagine it will be talked about throughout the village by the end of the day".

"Unfortunately", he continued, "as it was an official complaint I have to go through the whole process and submit a report". He then asked where I was from and when I said Newcastle, he looked startled again until I told him where I was staying and why.

He took George and Avril's address, which I actually remembered after a moment's panic. Imagine what he would have thought or done if I had forgotten it.

He left saying he thought the matter would go no further than submitting his report and with a smile and a wave he reversed back down the lane and that was the end of it or so I thought! I kept chuckling away to myself as I set off again down the lane to the river, thinking Rosalynde and Co would be amused when I told them about my "arrest" over breakfast.

About an hour later and without further incident I arrived back at the A69 and crossed over into the village. In defiance I walked in a true Qi Gong fashion back to the house and I couldn't help glancing at all the windows wondering who it was who had reported my "escape". I wondered what they thought if they recognized me as the reported "madman" and why I hadn't been escorted back to the "Garlands" by the police but there was no reaction from any of the houses.

I had quite a reception when I opened the door and stepped into the house. Everyone burst out laughing and I wondered how on earth they knew about my escapade. Rosalynde explained......

Apparently, with the sun streaming through the bedroom window she couldn't go back to sleep and decided to dress and do her exercises in the garden. She, too, had crept downstairs without disturbing anyone.

However, like me she couldn't find the front or back door keys and hadn't thought about climbing out of a window and started to do her exercises in the lounge. A short while later she heard a quiet tap on the front door and went to investigate thinking it was me. It is a frosted double glazed door and she could make out the outline of a man in a dark suit outside. Not wanting to wake anyone, she tried to speak through the glass explaining she couldn't find the key. The man must have understood her because he shouted "What about the back door?"

"I can't find that either", said Rosalynde beginning to feel rather foolish, and she tried to explain it wasn't her house and everyone else was asleep. The man didn't seem to understand and began pointing to the ground. Rosalynde began to get suspicious and started to back away towards the telephone. Then the figure, she still hadn't realized it was a policeman, suddenly seemed to bend double and sink to the ground. Rosalynde stopped, fascinated at this and wondered what he was going to do next. Then the letterbox, which was right at the bottom of the door, opened and a voice said "Halloooo!"

Rosalynde had forgotten about the letterbox being so low because of the large area of double glazing and waited expectantly.

"Halloooo", again then "Sorry to bother you but I'm a policeman making some enquiries about a gentleman who says he's staying here". Two fingers appeared in the gap holding a police warrant card.

"Oh God, it's George, what's happened now?" was her first thought. She quickly knelt down on the floor and placing her head on the threshold, found herself staring into the perplexed eyes of my young policeman, who must have had his head on the single step to be able to peer through the other side of the letterbox.

"Do you have a Mr George Walker staying with you?" was the policeman's first question.

"Yes", replied Rosalynde, "he's my husband".

I can imagine the policeman, after seeing me, thinking "I'm not surprised they seem well matched for each other", but like a good officer, he nodded (sideways) and continued the rather ludicrous conversation through the letterbox. Rosalynde at this point explained more carefully about the problem with the keys and had no idea where her sister, who was very security conscious, had hidden them.

"That's perfectly alright, madam" was the reply as though it was an everyday occurrence to question people six or so inches above the ground.

Fortunately, at that point, Avril, woken by the strange goings on, appeared on the scene in her dressing gown and after a quick explanation from Rosalynde, produced the key and opened the door as the policeman climbed stiffly to his feet and began brushing the dust off his knees and elbows, struggling at the same time to regain his dignity and bring a semblance of sanity to the situation. He was quickly invited in and after a cup of tea and slice of toast, during which time the whole story came out, the policeman closed his notebook, bade Rosalynde and Avril farewell and returned to his car probably wondering if it was going to continue being "one of those days!"

He then drove down the street, turned into the main road, saw me returning with my arms waving about, mounted the pavement in shock and ran over me before crashing into a garden wall, putting both of us in the Garlands Hospital (in adjacent beds) for a month; after which he stood trial for dangerous driving, lost his licence and was dismissed from the police force ……………….. only joking! I never saw him again but I bet he remembers me.

The whole episode took place in under an hour between 6 am and 7 am approximately. What a start to the day and who said "There's nothing funny about cancer!"?

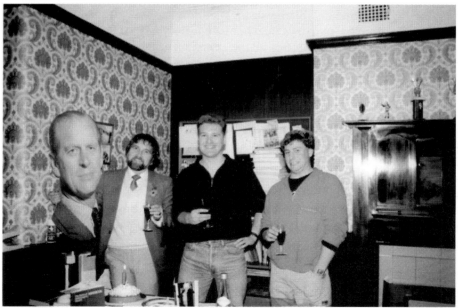

Celebrating the Duke of Edinburgh's Award Scheme's 30th Anniversary in my work office during happier and healthier times (before 1988) with Andy Brook & Roy Keegan, two of my staff

181

Chapter 43
Foot and Mouth and Another More Personal Crisis

We had a much happier Christmas and New Year than last year, ,which was marred by salmonella poisoning, the Freeman Hospital and what was to follow. Marc and Roxanne both came home and spent the festive season with us. Marc's partner had gone to France to be with her family and Roxanne's new partner, Phil, joined us when he could.

We were going to spend New Year's Eve at our cottage – we'd even kept some fireworks back from Guy Fawke's Night there to celebrate. Unfortunately, neither happened because we had very severe weather and decided to stay at home. As we all wished each other "Happy New Year" I couldn't help thinking, "I hope it was going to be just that", but deep down I wondered if it really was going to be the sort of year I had been hoping for, for so long now. A full, clear year always seemed to be the big hurdle and it was always around that time that something would go dreadfully wrong.

Marc and Roxanne seemed to be very happy. Marc's new job , which had brought him back from London to Edinburgh, was going well for him. His new firm, "Logica", an international information technology company, had sent him off on his first big challenge to Aberdeen where he was to work as a Consultant with the big oil company, Shell, for the next few months. It meant living in a hotel in Aberdeen for five days then home to Edinburgh for the weekend but he was really enjoying it and putting all the experience he had gained in London to the test.

Roxanne and her first partner, Russell, had separated after seven years but remained good friends. We were probably more upset than they were because we had come to like Russell very much and accepted him as part of our family. Russell has now fallen in love again and likewise with Roxanne, whose new young man, Phil, has many excellent attributes and a great sense of humour. Roxanne has been looking for a new job and seems, at last, to have found something, which I feel she will both enjoy and be good at – helping to look after the countryside and environment. It is still with a government ministry but it is a brand new department based very near Westerhope where she lives. She has always been a great supporter of anything which will benefit the planet; she loves animals and has always helped those people unfortunate enough to be struggling to survive in this sometimes very harsh world of ours. This new department is about to open and I'm sure it will become instantly embroiled in the recent, dreadful, foot and mouth disease, which has been causing great misery and distress to this country and none more so than our farming community. If that is the case Roxanne will have to steel herself to face the flood of tragic circumstances which she will encounter on a daily basis. Knowing her as I do she will cope and whoever she deals with will feel her empathy and understanding even over the telephone. Whatever happens I am very proud of both of them and love them very much.

As I am writing this chapter Easter is looming up on the horizon and there are even signs of spring as the weather has slowly started to change for the better. But what is sadly missing, as we drive around the roads and lanes of Northumberland, are the lambs which are usually gambolling in the fields at this time. The fields are empty, devoid of all creatures, great and small, and it is a constant reminder of how quickly and drastically things can go wrong even in this age of incredible scientific discovery. Just as poignant, however, are the clusters of farm building in the midst of these fields where there too seems to be no signs of life. Life there is, though, families of people temporarily isolated from the rest of society because of a disease which has gone out of control. People whose very livelihood is now threatened and whose future will need more than a miracle to help them reach the stability they had before things like BSE, foot and mouth and mountains of European Community beaurocracy landed on their shoulders.

We have a number of farmer friends but none more close than David and Marlyn Mair, who farm the land where our cottage is situated and, of course, Suzanne Manuell and her husband, William, who have a large diary farm in Cornwall.

Since the outbreak we have not visited our cottage, not wishing to risk the chance of introducing the disease, especially as we live very close to where the outbreak was supposed to have started. We obviously hope the cottage is surviving the elements, which have raged around there from time to time. So far, we know that David and Marlyn have escaped the disease but we know what they must have gone through day after day and our thoughts constantly go out to them. Similarly so with Suzanne and William, they have not been affected; that is not quite true, it is impossible not to be affected especially if you are a farmer. Their farm had already been hit by the severe drops in the price of milk before foot and mouth reared its ugly head. Suzanne had helped them survive this by developing a thriving bed and breakfast business on the farm but with the Easter holidays looming up she must be very worried about bookings.

Back here in Newcastle we were busy preparing for her sixth fundraising concert, which was showing all the signs of being another sell out. Underlying this, however, was the worry that if foot and mouth struck their farm, she couldn't possibly leave William, even for a weekend, to face the trauma and horror that would descend upon them.

Fortunately, it never came to that, she and Anthony Seddon, her brilliant and lovable accompanist, made it. Her special guest, James Cleverton, the young bass-baritone was an instant hit. He sang at our Millennium concert and later starred in Mozart's opera, "Cosi fan Tuti", produced and directed by Ben Luxon in Glasgow, which we were fortunate to see. This also turned out to be an even greater bonus for us. Only a couple of weeks earlier, I had received a telephone call from Sir Thomas Allen, which brought bad news. He was unable to sing for us at our Proms in October because of a change of circumstance. He had to perform in a special concert in Los Angeles, which had been cancelled freeing him to sing for us but it was now going ahead and he could not back out of it. What could I say? Tom had already given us three fantastic concerts, which were more than I had ever dared hope. His arrival on the "team" could not have come at a more opportune time, especially with Ben Luxon's tragic hearing problems. Of course, I was deeply disappointed and I sensed that Tom was too but my "cancer-training" came to the fore. I had faced disappointments before and Tom's promise to sing for us next year was the measure of the man and I knew we had enough success and support to survive a year without him. Something would turn up and it did in the form of a tall, dark haired, bearded young man who, only a few days before Suzanne's concert, returned from a successful tour of South Africa with Broomhill Opera, a prestigious London-based opera company. The production was Bizet's Carmen, in which he had one of the principal roles.

By the end of the first half of our concert I'd made up my mind. Turning to Richard Bloodworth and Len Young, the conductors, who had conducted our Proms since the very first performance in 1990 and who were sitting behind me, I mouthed "What do you think?" They knew about Tom as we'd had an emergency meeting and I had suggested they listen to Jim as a possible replacement for Tom, young though he was. Richard mouthed back "Book him" and Len nodded in agreement. I slipped out of the auditorium and up to the dressing room, where I told our three stars for the evening what a great first half it had been and the audience was buzzing about it. I then told Jim about the Proms and asked him if he would like to join the "team" for this year's concert. He said he would love to and we shook hands on it.

When I introduced the second half, I announced just that and there was an instant burst of applause from an audience, which obviously wholeheartedly approved and I could see that Jim was very moved by the response.

We had another first that evening too, after several years of fruitless attempts to persuade Anthony to play a solo piece on the piano, he finally acquiesced. He even addressed the audience, who actually heard him speak for the first time in six years, and told them that under great duress and after dire threats of what I had told him I would do to certain private parts of his anatomy, he was about to give a solo performance of "Marigold" by Billy Mayerl. He then proceeded to enthrall everyone with that lovely, light, sparkling tune. When he finished he looked across at me and smiled and I returned the smile with both thumbs held up in the air.

It was another wonderful evening and I've added it to the other 22 (I think) wonderful evenings Rosalynde and I have produced together with more than a little help from our fantastic, musical friends. Oh yes, I nearly forgot we raised over £6,400.00 and £400.00 of that was donated by people who couldn't attend but wanted to contribute anyway. Where else does that sort of generosity and support exist?

Throughout the weeks of planning and apart from the tragedy of the foot and mouth and Tom Allen's withdrawal from the Proms, there was only one other cloud hanging over us and it was my old enemy breaking into my life again. Nothing untoward that I had discovered during my own regular body checks but a feeling of misgiving brought about by a loss of appetite again and body weight, which is always cause for concern. I was finding that my low tolerance to warm temperatures was also bothering me again and I would sweat a lot during the day, especially in the mornings and if I was exerting myself physically. I've never suffered from night sweats which is often caused by lymphoma, so that eased my mind a little but I spent regular, uncomfortable moments during the day, which made me worry. Rosalynde was the opposite and always felt the cold so we had constant but friendly clashes over opening and closing windows, lowering and raising the central heating temperature and so on. I was also still experiencing chest palpitations and headaches but had learned to live with both as all the tests proved negative and stress was given as the likely cause. I also suffered from, sometimes severe, stomach pains in the area of the two major operations carried out in 1988 and 1989. These were caused by scar tissue forming and could be very unpleasant at times. It must read as though I am turning into a hypochondriac but I'm not. This is what I have to put up with as the price of remaining alive all this time. It does affect my life and constantly reminds me of my immortality and it also has its affect on Rosalynde, who has had to carry the brunt of all my moments of pain, anguish, fear and depression. But, she has never faltered and constantly reminds me of the good feelings she always has about the future. Bless you, Rosalynde, for your love, your courage, your steadfastness and for just being you, the girl I fell in love with all those years ago. I sometimes feel I don't deserve this devotion because of all the bad times I have pulled you into but my life has been enriched because of you.

The situation at this present moment is that my last two check ups at the RVI showed nothing sinister except that one of the blood tests on both occasions indicated the possibility of lymphoma activity. It could also indicate other things too but the uncertainty was now there. I had a third blood test two weeks ago but have surprisingly heard nothing about it and I've been reluctant to chase it up in case the news isn't encouraging.

The combination of all these facts has resulted in an appointment for a full, upper body scan scheduled for 18 April 2001 and I will receive the results on 25 April 2001 – another long, awful wait. I also discovered something very disturbing about scanning when the decision was made for me to have one. Apparently, a scan is equivalent to approximately 90 x-rays and that is the first time in 12 years that I have been told that! I couldn't believe it and was shocked at the news. I can't remember how many CT scans I've had but it must be between 12 and 15, which means I've had the equivalent of between 1,080 and 1,350 x-rays, not counting the many normal x-rays I've had too. The cost to my physical well-being over these years has been very high and in more ways than one. I'm amazed at how my body is still functioning and where on earth I've found the drive and energy to organize all those concerts on top of everything else, during all that time. No wonder I have to fight, sometimes daily, to appear normal to my family and friends. No wonder I sometimes feel it would be easier just to give up and let the worst happen.

The biggest test of all will take place on 25th April when I find out the CT scan results. If they are clear then I have to carry on as usual and try to overcome the debilitating effects of all these side effects. If it is not then a whole new ball game is placed before me; a game which will have frightening possibilities. Another occurrence of the illness will be added to an already large number and each recurrence lessens the chance of an outright win. Treatment options are still available but are also running out. I certainly do not want to go through another year like last year and if that is the only option then I will probably say "That's it, enough is enough". Believe me, I have thought long and hard about this very possibility and somehow I will find the strength to make the right decision.

I have a lot to lose, everything in fact. I have had many wonderful moments since 1988 most of them brought about by cancer and I keep telling myself that I could have died that year and several other times since but I didn't for all the reasons I have written about. So in many ways I've been very lucky and certainly so because of people like Rosalynde, Marc, Roxanne, Ben & Sheila Luxon, Tom Allen, Janice Cairns, Suzanne Manuel, the late Derrick Phoenix, Richard Bloodworth, Len Young, Steve Proctor, Peter Carey, our very close friends and on and on and on. The list is endless and I want them all to know how much their love and friendship has meant to me, not just in the good times but in the dark times too.

I said in my opening address at Suzanne's last concert that there are only two real Kingdom's on this planet – the Kingdom of the Sick and the Kingdom of the Healthy. Everyone of us carries two passports – one for each Kingdom. We must all endeavour to remain in the Kingdom of the Healthy at all costs and to do this we must help ourselves and help each other without fail – a daunting task when you realize how much disease and illness exist around us and, sadly, some of it self-inflicted.

I didn't want to end this chapter on a low note so here is the bright side. Rosalynde and I have just booked a holiday and cruise around the Canary Islands and North Africa. We leave on Friday, returning over the Easter weekend. It was a spur of the moment decision and we are going to enjoy it and forget about scans, hospital visits, concert organization etc, until we get back. Five days after that I will have the scan and a week after that my results.

What the hell, if they are good, fantastic! If they are not so good, Rosalynde and I will face them as we've done many times in the past, together, and still make some plans for the future.

One question is bugging me, however, which takes me back to the Freeman Hospital about this time last year when Steve Proctor broke the bad news to me. It is the same question I asked him then.

"Do I pay my bloody golf fees this year?"

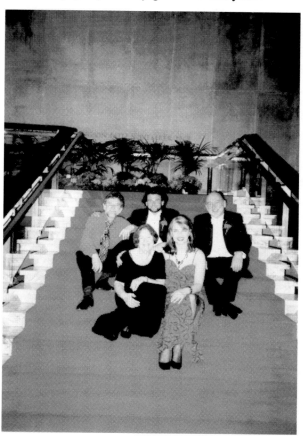

Suzanne & Anthony's
special guest,
James Cleverton
(April 2001)

Chapter 44
The Showdown

The cruise I mentioned at the end of the last chapter rapidly loomed up and we were both looking forward to this long awaited and much needed break. Only one thing was marring it for me but I didn't tell Rosalynde as I did not wish to spoil this for her in any way and that was my loss of appetite. I knew from past experience that food on cruise ships was usually excellent and in great abundance and I could see that becoming a real problem. As luck would have it, I was sorting out my wash bag and various medicines I thought would be necessary for the trip (Steve had already provided me with some antibiotics in case of emergency) and I came across a bottle containing seven Dexamethasone tablets (a steroid used to pick you up and stimulate appetite amongst other things). These were some of the tablets which Steve had stopped when I went through the blind and deaf episode before Christmas and I hadn't resumed any of them.

I had a short battle of conscience, arguing that I would have had them anyway and I would "confess my sins" to Steve on my return. That decided me and I started on one a day as prescribed on the bottle. It gave me two days before the cruise and five days on, by then the tablets and the sea air should hopefully do the trick.

After the usual, hectic packing and making sure everything we left behind was organized for our return, which meant a long list of things for our daughter, Roxanne, who was beginning to realize she was living too near home for comfort!

We flew from Newcastle Airport to Tenerife, which is always a godsend for northerners, and we joined the ship about 8 hours later linking up with our friends, John and Catherine Baugh. They were waiting for us as we boarded and Catherine, always the great organizer, rushed us off to find our cabin and here we had a most amazing stroke of luck. They had booked their cruise over a year earlier and ours was just a last minute decision and, incredibly, with all the hundreds of cabins on the ship at five different levels our cabin was just around the corner from there's, about six rooms away. As Richard Meldrew would have said "I don't believe it!" except his cabin would have been 600 cabins away and five decks down.

We had a great holiday, weather was good and we visited Madiera, Morocco, Gran Canaria and Lanzarote, finally returning to Tenerife where we left the Baughs, who were having an extra week on the island. We promised to see them again for some more golf, caravanning and cycling in the summer.

Arriving in Newcastle in the early hours of the morning soon brought us back down to earth (excuse the pun) and we were quickly conditioning ourselves to a cold, north eastern, Easter Bank Holiday weekend but the memories lingered on and we both felt refreshed and more alive than we had done earlier.

Appetite-wise, steroids, fresh sea air and relaxation had seemed to have done the trick and I desperately hoped that things were on the turn and all my worrying had proved groundless. However, as the days went by my appetite slowly started to deteriorate. On top of that my CT scan was due on the Wednesday after the Easter week and so that didn't help matters.

I have mentioned this several times in both my books that probably the worst thing of all is the "waiting game". If you allow it, and it's so easy to do so, things can quickly spiral out of control.; cracks appear, the imagination starts running riot and you start being very afraid. Strangely enough, once the facts are known and provided the situation revealed is not the "end of the world" then something else takes over inside and slowly you regain control of your life and start working towards removing the obstacle course you have been struggling to overcome. I've come through this cycle many times now and I only hope that if things go wrong again this time I will somehow find the strength to win through again.

Of one thing I am sure, if there is a way Steve Proctor will find it and I have no worries about the love and support I will receive from Rosalynde, Marc and Roxanne and everyone else involved in helping me in my fight to survive. Those ingredients are vital to the survival of anyone struggling with a life threatening disease.

Wednesday arrived and I had my scan – at the General Hospital this time not the RVI so once again I had run a complete circle to the beginning of it all in 1988. I looked for "Charlie Bear" the symbol of the first Charlie Bear Scan Appeal in the scan room and there he was, my old friend of nearly 14 years now!

It usually takes a week to receive the results so the waiting game has to continue. Sometimes the results have come through quickly for me and Steve has on occasions been able to ring me earlier and put my mind at rest. This, unfortunately, can create a dilemma in an already over-wraught imagination and the sequence can be like this:-

a)   if the results are early and they are good an early message is wonderful.

b)   But... once this process starts it can turn around on you e.g. what if the results were not   good would it help to make earlier contact or better to wait for the appropriate appointment?

You can see the quandary which can manifest itself. This happened to me; Steve was away at a conference and I heard nothing up till the day of the appointment. That morning a letter arrived from the RVI which I opened with great trepidation. It informed me that due to reorganisation my appointment for the following morning had been put back a fortnight. I groaned inwardly and showed it to Rosalynde.

"What the hell do I do now?" I moaned.

One Lump or Two

"There's only one thing you can do", was Rosalynde's expected and practical reply "Ring the hospital and explain the predicament".

I hesitated because by this time I had almost convinced myself that, with not hearing early, the results were not going to be good. All I was doing was burying my head in the sand, of course, but that is the way it becomes.

"I'll think about it", I said " and will probably ring this afternoon". I knew Rosalynde had to go out so I thought it would be best then and if things were against me, it would give me time to compose myself before breaking the news to her.

As it turned out, I didn't have to ring the hospital. A nurse on Ward 8 where I have received most of my treatment rang me to pass on a message from Professor Proctor to inform me that he was unable to see me on Wednesday as arranged but would be in touch as soon as he returned from his London conference. That was a relief as obviously he hadn't yet seen the results so I took the chance while I had it and explained to the nurse about the awaited scan results. She was very sympathetic and said she'd do her best to see if one of the doctors could track them down for me and contact me.

About 30 plus hours later, on the Wednesday afternoon, when I was frantically trying to do things to take my mind of it the telephone rang............ I recognized the calm, professional but friendly voice immediately – it was Steve Proctor.

I felt a surge of great relief flow over me when he then said,

"Your scan results are clear – absolutely great news, I'm very pleased for you. There's obviously something else causing the pains in your stomach area and also affecting your appetite. We'll sort things out next time I see you. I gather your appointment has been changed to a fortnight – we'll leave things till then. In the meantime try taking some antacids and let me know if they make any improvement – I suspect there may be an ulcer lurking around down there".

I never made that appointment; by the end of the following week, the pain and loss of appetite grew steadily worse and in the end I had no other alternative but to ask Rosalynde to ring Ward 8 and explain my predicament.

The response, as usual, was immediate and I was told to attend the new Haematology Department (Ward 6a) next to Ward 8 for an appointment.

It was very busy when we arrived there and eventually I saw Dr Anne Lennard, who has seen me on more than one occasions when Steve was away at various meetings. She did her usual thorough examination and asked all the pertinent questions. At the end of it she shook her head and said "Well, with your excellent scan results this doesn't make sense to me and I'm lost for an answer".

This was unusual for Anne so I waited expectantly. "I've got all your notes and will talk to Steve about this as soon as he returns which I think is sometime tomorrow. Meanwhile if the pain becomes difficult take some soluble paracetamol. Don't worry we'll get to the bottom of it".

My next visit to the RVI was, of course, with Steve and after another extensive body check, he talked earnestly to Rosalynde and myself answering our many questions at the same time. He was obviously concerned about my stomach and possible bowel problem where the pain seemed to circulate between the two areas, which were adjacent anyway.

"I think the best thing to do under the circumstances", he concluded "will be to book you into Ward 8 where we'll keep a bed for you on a day to day basis, depending of course, on how busy the ward is, and we'll put you through a number of tests which should help me to sort this out".

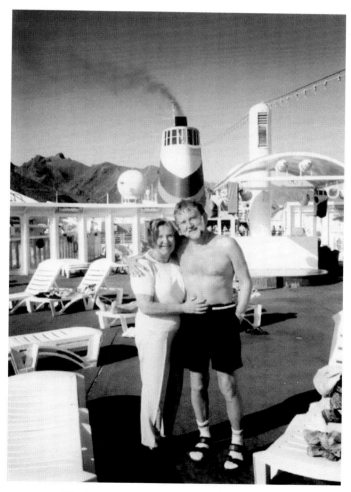

The last minute cruise - Canaries & North Africa

Chapter 45
Ward 8 and Luxury

Two days later I was back on Ward 8 and followed this up by having a new hospital experience. It turned out the room I was having was needed for an emergency and there wasn't another bed available. It looked as though I would have to go back home and wait but within about 20 minutes Lorna Renwick appeared and said they'd found me a bed in Bishop Ward just down the corridor. She had a twinkle in her eye as she said "It's a private ward but Steve has a special arrangement if we have problems and they have a spare room".

It was only 50 yards down the corridor and a couple of minutes later Rosalynde and I were ushered into a luxurious reception area and taken down the carpetted corridor into a side room. It was quite something, spacious, beautifully carpeted and curtained and another door led into the en-suite bathroom.

The only thing which spoilt the few days I was there, was that I could not eat, or very little of, the excellent food the chef kept tempting me with.

This was no mass produced, heated, trolley delivery of mundane, National Health Service fayre; it was cooked in the ward's own kitchen by a trained chef, who popped into your room about an hour before a meal offering you a choice of "goodies" which would not have disgraced a popular, high standard restaurant and which sadly I could barely face, nevermind eat!

The nursing staff were excellent too and always popping in to chat and see if I needed anything. During my stay there the process of solving my health setback began in earnest.

I was visited daily by the doctors from Ward 8, checked thoroughly and told what was going to happen. Firstly, they had to bring the pain under control and then the test would begin. At first I was given two painkillers every six hours but between these times the pain would occasionally become worse so I was given a liquid painkiller, which contained a tiny percentage of morphine and that gave me great relief.

As well as the bowel and stomach area being in great discomfort, I was also finding it difficult to breathe without panting every time I exerted myself, even just walking along the ward corridor for exercise. I became really worried because the symptoms were similar to the salmonella poisoning in the lungs last year – had some of it survived the lung, clean out operation and after lying dormant for over a year had suddenly sprung to activity again? The doctors did not think so but I was sent for an x-ray as a precaution and a small shadow of infection was found instead. Antibiotics were administered and it slowly cleared up but at this present moment I'm still being affected by it; probably because of my very weakened condition. My few days of being pampered came to an end and I was transferred back to Ward 8 as they had a room there available for me.

During the next few days I went through a planned series of tests and probably the most important one of all was the endoscopy. This was my second experience of this particular medical test. I'd had one in November 2000 when it really all began. Steve had described it to me, also telling me he had gone through it himself months earlier and there was a choice. As a miniature camera is fed through the mouth, down the gullet into the stomach, it is obviously very uncomfortable so if you wish you can be sedated and it is "painless". Steve said he had not opted for sedation but experienced it the "hard" way.

"It can't be all that bad then", I had thought so I opted to do it in the "macho" way when my appointment arrived. It was an experience and although not painful it was uncomfortable and what was really embarrassing was the explosion of air which seemed to roar out of my mouth. I sounded like a elephant with a bad attack of the wind! The nurse was holding me and encouraged me in a gentle, firm and quiet voice, while the doctor probed the camera around my stomach. I was able to watch the whole process on the monitor screen and could clearly see the tube with the tiny camera attached to its end!   It only lasts about five minutes but it seemed longer and when the camera was finally withdrawn the doctor told me he had taken a small scraping for biopsy.

The results showed everything was normal but the biopsy had revealed the presence of helicobacter pylori in the stomach. For years the medical world did not think that bugs of any kind could survive in the acids produced by the stomach but a few years ago an Australian researcher did, in fact, discover the one mentioned above, also known as H Pylori for short. This little "devil" manifests itself in childhood and can slowly produce ulcers over the years. Since this amazing discovery the bug can be easily wiped out with a course of antibiotics and that's the end of it.   This discovery has changed many people's lives and has saved hospitals millions of pounds over the years. One other grizzly effect it can have but fortunately this is rare, is that if left undetected and untreated it can trigger off lymphoma activity in the stomach and bowel areas. Apparently I had no ulcers and after a week's prescribed course of the appropriate drugs I was rid of it forever.

Several months later I had my second endoscopy but this time I opted for the sedation and can't remember a thing about it. Anne Lennard appeared in my room a few days later with my file and results and dropped the bad news as gently as she could.

"There are ulcers in the stomach lining", she explained and proceeded to show me two (I think) colour photographs of them and they looked awful, one was bleeding.

"Well ulcers are ulcers", I thought, "but they can be treated".

"I've seen ulcers like this many times", Anne said in a quiet voice, "and I'm sorry to tell you that these have all the signs of being caused by lymphoma".

One Lump or Two

The shock waves hit me but I tried hard to put on a brave face and began tentatively asking her questions.

"We have to wait for the biopsy results and Steve should be back from his conference trip by then so I'll discuss all this with him and we'll set off from there". She left and I just laid back on my bed and slowly watched the ceiling and walls close in as though to either crush me or wrap themselves around me in a form of defensive curtain, I wasn't quite sure.

I didn't mention anything to Rosalynde for a couple of days and then when I was told that Steve had returned and would see me in the morning, I explained everything to her on her evening visit beforehand. I saw the pain in her eyes for a brief moment but then it vanished and she said in a strong voice.

"Bugger! Bugger! Bugger! After all you've been through and now this". I've never heard Rosalynde so unladylike but her anger helped me to continue with the details. I told her Steve was seeing me in the morning and I really wanted her to be there when he did – I needed her strength and incredible optimism once again. The meeting took place and Lorna Renwick joined us with Steve.

"The biopsy has confirmed lymphoma but the good news is that it is low grade and it appears to be contained in the stomach area although I still need to check the bowel area nearby just in case. There is no sign of the disease in the spleen, kidneys or liver so that is also very favourable. I know when we talked last year when I had to hit you hard with a drug regime that you said you would not go through that again if it ever came back and I respect that. I have, however, gone over your history and I want to put you onto a drug you've never had before, which is normally used for Hodgkin's Lymphoma whereas yours is non-Hodgkin's lymphoma. It has been tried successfully with patients similar to yourself. The side effects are reasonably minimal, 48 hours sickness but you don't lose your hair".

He went on to explain that I would be given three tablets and various anti-sickness tablets, plus other pills to counteract infections because my immune system would be weakened again. These three tablets worked in the body for four weeks and then I would have another three. Tests would be carried out to see the results. After that he would have to take things from there.

After Steve and Lorna left the room Rosalynde and I talked about Steve's summary of it all and we felt better for it. Rosalynde had to dash so I was left on my own to think things over. The door opened and Lorna reappeared. She came over and sat on my bed, put her arms around me and gave me a big hug and whispered in my ear "You are a wonderful man, you know, I don't think you realize how many people you have helped and how much pleasure you have given with your concerts. The drug Steve mentioned is very good – we'll get you through".

I was very moved by her words and felt a choking in my throat and tears forming in my eyes. I managed to control myself but I'm sure Lorna was aware of my emotion as she hugged me even tighter.

After she left I thought about how I was going to break the news to Marc and Roxanne. Marc was coming home from Edinburgh for the weekend. I wasn't keen on telling them as they had enough to worry about but Rosalynde insisted they would be very hurt if I didn't.

On the Saturday, Rosalynde, Marc and Roxanne visited me at the hospital and I took the "bull by the horns" and told them all the news emphasizing the encouraging details given to me by Steve.

Shortly after they left Steve popped into see me and said I could go home for the rest of the weekend and return on Monday morning. That was a real bonus and as the weather was very warm and sunny we spent most of Sunday sitting in the garden.

On the Monday evening I had my first chemotherapy – the three capsules I mentioned earlier backed up with anti-sickness pills. I had a restless night and although feeling nauseous most of the time I wasn't sick and things slowly started to improve. On the following Monday I received the good news that I could go home and, unless there were any complications, I could have my final checks, which would consist of an ultrasound scan of the abdomen followed by a CT scan of the same area. A barium meal was planned for the day after then I would report to Steve Proctor in the afternoon of 26th May for the results and whatever was to happen to me next – my life in his hands!

The two days it took were harrowing for me bringing back all sorts of memories, most of them best forgotten especially the injections, which I was beginning to dread, as my veins were affected by the many punctures they had sustained.

The barium meal on the second day took ages. A white fluid has to be drunk then successive x-rays are taken as the liquid moves through the bowels. Some people take longer than others usually two to four hours but on very rare occasions it can take up to a week – the mind boggles at that!

My appointment with Steve Proctor at 2 pm that afternoon had to be put on hold and it looked as though I would have to see him on another day – another extended worrying wait for the results. As luck would have it (good luck for a change) the barium meal passed through in three hours and I was able to see Steve. I was not looking forward to it and as I sat waiting for him to see me all the doubts and fears kept running through my mind – had it spread, was this the end of the line! Fortunately, I didn't have all that long to wait and Steve called me into his consulting room. He was smiling and I thought that was a good omen and cheered up.

First he gave my abdomen area a thorough check, commenting how thin I was but that would help his examination. He was pleased with the results and after I dressed he proceeded to bring me up to date except for the last two days of tests. It was all very encouraging and I mentally heaved a sigh of relief – hope was back. He then moved to the plan for the future.

"From this point in time", he began, "we move to get everything under control. You'll continue with this drug, which still has two weeks to go then we'll repeat it and do some checks. After that I'm considering putting you on an immune booster such as Levamisole or Interferon.

I listened intently and he continued "I've been having discussions with Graham Jackson and he's been doing some research into some very interesting and encouraging results from the drug, Thalidomide; you remember it was used as a sedative for pregnant woman with catastrophic damage to the babies who were born badly deformed. Although it is a "banned" drug it has been used for other treatments and considerable research has and is being done on it. From our point of view they have discovered that Thalidomide combined with a steroid has had amazing results on tumours including lymphoma. I intend to consider putting you on this after you've finished this treatment. This "cocktail" has so far shown minimal side effects"

When he had finished I felt the hope grow even stronger and after he gave me a prescription for various tablets I would need over the next few weeks and thanked him for once again injecting me with the "Proctor tonic".

Back home I broke the news to Rosalynde and we hugged each other with relief.

And this is where the story ends but there will be an epilogue and I have paid my golf fees for this year!!

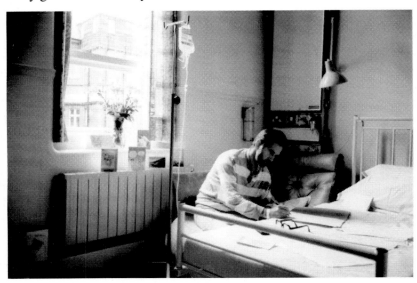

Determined to finish this book - even in hospital !

196

Epilogue

During all these events two things occurred which brought a ray of sunshine into my rather bleak but improving situation.

The first was a letter from London thanking me for money we had raised and given to the Bristol Cancer Centre during the last 10 years. It was signed Richard (Briers) and I began to wonder if it could possibly be the Richard Briers of the "Good Life" and, more recently, "Monarch of the Glen". I wrote back thanking him and asked him if, in fact, he was and a few days later another letter arrived from him with a picture postcard of Glen Bogle with the key characters superimposed on it. His note cleared up the mystery and I was very impressed by the fact that such a busy, famous man could go to the bother to actually contact me in such a friendly way.

The other surprise happened on the Monday morning when I was due to return to the RVI to start chemotherapy and I was feeling very low. The post arrived just as we were leaving and we began opening it; we receive many, many letters during the year and especially at ticket booking time for the Proms Concert, which was actually only a couple of weeks away. I picked up a large brown envelope addressed to me with "Strictly Confidential" on it and then I noticed the words "From the Prime Minister". This really puzzled me and I hesitatingly opened it and read the contents.

It said that the Prime Minister wished to submit my name to the Queen to graciously ask her if she would be agreeable to honour me with the Award of the Member of the Order of the British Empire (M.B.E.)

I was dumbfounded and handed it to Rosalynde who, after reading it, gave me a big hug and said, "What a wonderful surprise and after all you have done you really deserve it, I'm very proud of you".

These two surprises really helped me through the next few weeks and I often wondered who or how many people were involved in recommending me for this prestigious honour.

The only frustrating thing about it was I couldn't tell anyone except, of course, Rosalynde, Marc and Roxanne, which I did, feeling very proud when I saw the expressions on their faces. It also helped them to cope with the bad news, which I had given them about my situation.

The sequence of events, which follows the submission of the award to the Queen for approval, is that you hear nothing more from Downing Street until the Honours List is published, which in my case would be Saturday, 16 June 2001. Twelve hours before midnight on the Friday, lists are distributed to various newspapers and TV stations if they wish to contact people for their features. No mention could be made until after midday on Friday, 15 June 2001.

The final sheet in the Prime Minister's letter was to be signed by the nominee stating that he/she would be agreeable to accept the award if the Queen approved

– all very grand and mysterious.

Later that day I was given the three tablets of chemotherapy – three small, blue tablets which were, hopefully, going to bring things back to normality. Over the next 3-4 weeks I came to realize just how strong those tablets were.

The forecasted 48 hours of nausea was relatively mild but that was because of the anti-sickness tablets, which controlled it. It was the slow, weakening effect on my body, particularly the feet and lower legs, which was probably worsened by the loss of weight and body muscle during the spell when I couldn't eat. However, once the nausea had settled down Steve said I could go home and report back regularly for blood tests as platelets and haemoglobin would all drop over the next fortnight or so.

It was really great to be home and I slowly began to pick up my appetite and enjoy eating food again.

The steroids I was on made me extra hyperactive of course and I soon embarked on a very ambitious project of re-designing our garden at the back of the house. It is quite a large garden and I decided it was going to be as work free as I could make it. Something we could sit in and enjoy rather than forever growing vegetables and battling the elements and pests to see them survive.

Another reason for this burst of energy and enthusiasm is that it is our Ruby Wedding Anniversary on 12 August this year and I wanted to do something very special for Rosalynde which would always remind us of the 40 years of being together through thick and thin.

I was enthusiastically supported in this venture by John Gibson, a friend, who had been helping me with the garden work since last year when I was unable to do it myself. He was a godsend and between us the whole design began to take shape and run to schedule.

During this busy period of planning and hospital visits another of those interesting "out of the blue" occurrences took place.

On impulse Rosalynde and I drove up to the Railway Inn at Fourstone, situated about four miles outside of Hexham on the North Tyne. Our friends, Malcolm and Rebecca Readman, who had run the Red Lion at Milfield near our cottage, had recently bought it and they offered excellent food and beer. We also arranged to meet two other friends, Barry and Joyce there for lunch. As we were about to start eating a group of people came into the bar where we were seated. Four were young men and looked like technicians of sort, the other two were a more mature man and woman. They both looked artistically inclined. The woman intrigued me because I had a feeling I recognized her and more so when she came over to the table and said with a smile, "Your fish looks good, can you recommend it?" I did, because it was delicious and she returned to the bar. I leaned forward and whispered to my companions, "I'm sure that is Susannah York". I was pleasantly surprised when they all agreed I could be right.

There was only one way to find out and the opportunity arose when the older man left the bar and the younger men took their drinks to a table leaving "Susannah York" on her own. I stood up, much to Rosalynde's embarrassment as she knew full well what I was up to, and walked over to her.

"I'm sorry to bother you but are you by any chance Susannah York?" I blurted out.

"I might be" she replied with a smile I recognized immediately from seeing it light up the screen many times in her films.

We chatted briefly after that and I was able to tell her how much I had admired her work over the years. It turned out she was performing in a play at the Theatre Royal in Newcastle and they had slipped into the country for a break. I was very impressed with her pleasant, friendly attitude to a curious stranger who, in a way was interrupting her privacy, which must have happened many times over the years of being a famous actress and film star.

Back at the hospital Steve Proctor was very pleased at the response I was having with the chemotherapy. The pain in the stomach and bowel area was clearing up and the swelling went down, a tiny node which had appeared under my arm had also disappeared – all very good and encouraging news, and it did a great deal to boost my morale.

Then on the Friday afternoon of the 16 June, David Whetstone, the Arts and Entertainment Editor of the Journal rang Rosalynde (I was having a hospital check up) and told her that the Honours List had arrived and I had been awarded an M.B.E., the citation reading, "for services to the North East Promenaders Against Cancer Charity & Trust".

Rosalynde gave me the news as soon as I returned home and it was an absolutely thrilling moment for me. Everything seemed to happen at double speed after that and continued like that over the rest of the weekend and the following week.

A photographer from the Journal arrived first and our photograph appeared in the newspaper the next day. This must have triggered off a reaction because our phone never stopped ringing from people wanting to congratulate us.

The weekend itself couldn't have been better timed because it was also Father's Day on the Sunday. Marc and Catherine arrived from Edinburgh and along with Roxanne and Phil, we all went out for a celebratory meal to a lovely old country pub called the Robin Hood, about 14 miles from Westerhope.

It was a weekend I will never ever forget and I know now that it was due to a huge amount of hard work behind the scenes by many people who felt strongly enough that the work done by our charity, N.E.P.A.C., deserved recognition and I wish that everyone involved and especially Rosalynde could have had an award, not just me.

One Lump or Two

While I am writing this I am sitting in Ward 6a, the new Haematology Centre, having a blood transfusion, which is the result of further treatment I have been recently undergoing.

Unfortunately the "3 pills" treatment did not work or rather, did not fully work. It did, however, show that the lymphoma was still sensitive to chemotherapy but it would have to be a stronger concoction and ideally one that I hadn't been treated with before.

Professor Proctor discussed this with Rosalynde and me and told us he had a different drug to use, which had very good results but it had side effects one of which was some loss of hair again.

Rosalynde and I had already discussed this possibility as Steve had previously warned us that the "3 pills" treatment had only about 30% success with non-Hodgkins lymphoma. I hated the idea of hair loss again and wasn't sure whether I could take another series of strong, debilitating drugs and all the follow-up treatment that went with it.

We both came to the same conclusion that I still had so much to live for and I should give it another try.

I began the treatment over a week ago. This consisted of 5 daily, short injections of a drug which "opened the way", for want of a better description, for the last different drug injection, which took six hours to be fed into the bloodstream. This was the cancer-killing drug and the one, which caused the side effects and other damage to the body, particularly the bloodstream.

And so, here I am having blood and platelet transfusions because my red blood cells, white cells, haemoglobin and platelets are dangerously low and I am at serious risk from all sorts of injections, some of which can spread very rapidly through the body.

The next few weeks are going to be a bit of a nightmare. I know because I have been through it all before but our 40th Wedding Anniversary is in a couple of weeks' time, the 12th North East Last Night of the Proms is on 20th October, our trip to Buckingham Palace to meet the Queen for the presentation of my M.B.E. is expected soon, I want to pay my golf fees next year and last but not least I would miss all those people I love very much - my family and friends.

To all of you, who read this book and are affected in some way by whatever form of cancer, which has entered your lives, my closing words are that you must always and I repeat, always think in exactly the same way.

Footnote: Her Majesty, The Queen, presented me with the MBE on Monday 15th October at Buckingham Palace. Rosalynde, Marc & Roxanne were present - a very proud moment for all of us.

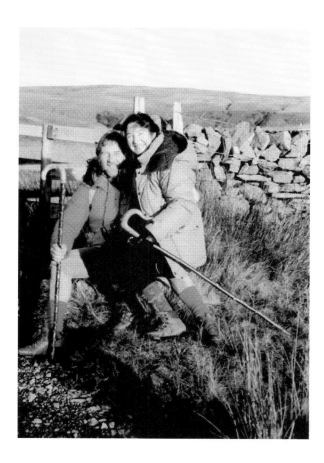

Still together
& very happy
after 40 Years

For a change -
everyone is smiling
at the same time

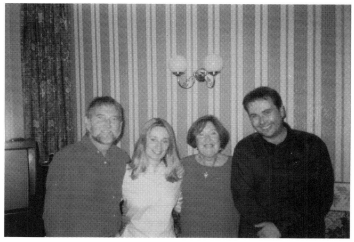

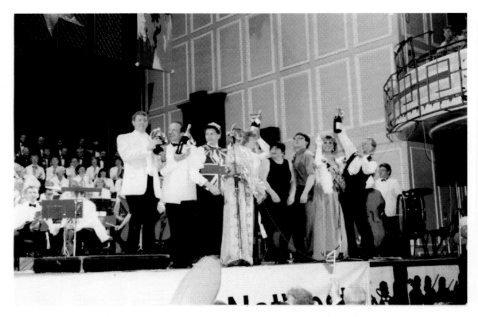

Celebrating the Proms (Champagne donated by Michael Jobling Wines, Newcastle)

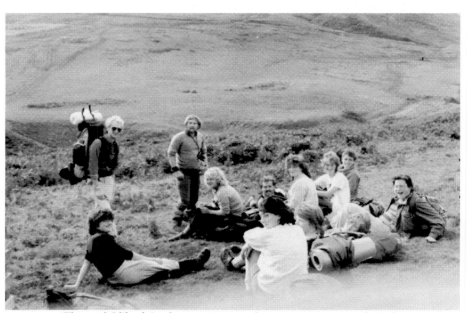

*The work I like doing best - training and assessing young people in the
Duke of Edinburgh Award Expedition Section*

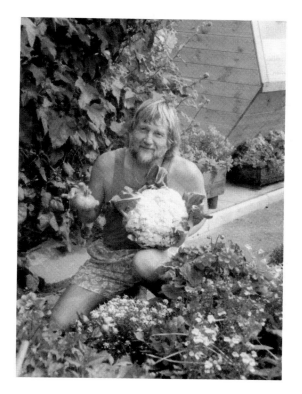

"Organic Gardener
of the Year"

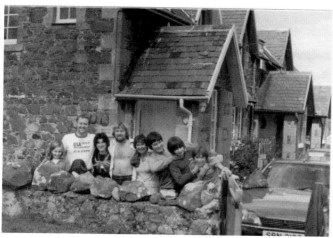

The Walker and Luxton Families at our cottage in 1977. A very young
Rachel Luxton, who is now singing in the Proms, would not look at the
camera! Ben was starring in the opera "Wozzeck" (Scottish Opera) at
Edinburgh at the time.

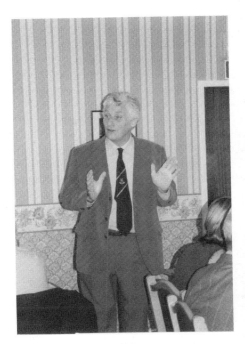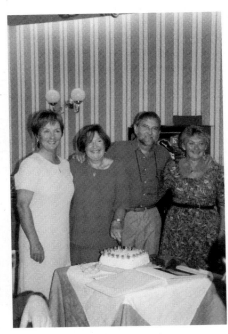

Left:The Best Man Right: The Bridesmaids

Below: Finally made it our 40th Wedding Anniversary - 12th August 2001 (The Family Table)

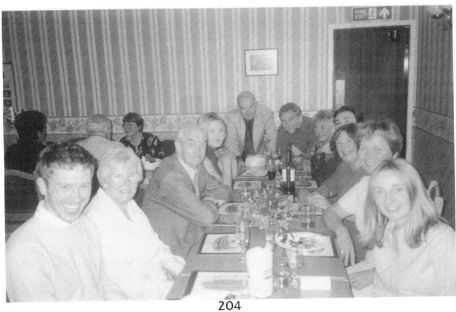